YOGA
for a Broken Heart

YOGA
for a Broken Heart

*A Spiritual Guide to Healing from
Break-up, Loss, Death or Divorce*

Michelle Paisley

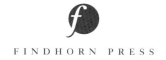

FINDHORN PRESS

© Michelle Paisley 2007

The right of Michelle Paisley to be identified as the author
of this work has been asserted by her in accordance
with the Copyright, Designs and Patents Act 1998.

First published in 2007 by Findhorn Press

ISBN 978-1-84409-114-0

All rights reserved.

The contents of this book may not be reproduced in
any form, except for short extracts for quotation or review,
without the written permission of the publisher.

Edited by Magaer Lennox

Cover design by Damian Keenan

Text design by The Bridgewater Book Company

Printed and bound by WS Bookwell, Finland

1 2 3 4 5 6 7 8 9 10 11 12 13 12 11 10 09 08 07

Published by

Findhorn Press

305a The Park, Findhorn

Forres IV36 3TE

Scotland, UK

Telephone +44-(0)1309-690582

Fax +44-(0)1309-690036

info@findhornpress.com

www.findhornpress.com

Dedication

To my daughters, my muses, who have taught me the meaning
of deep, unconditional, fearless trust and true love.

Contents

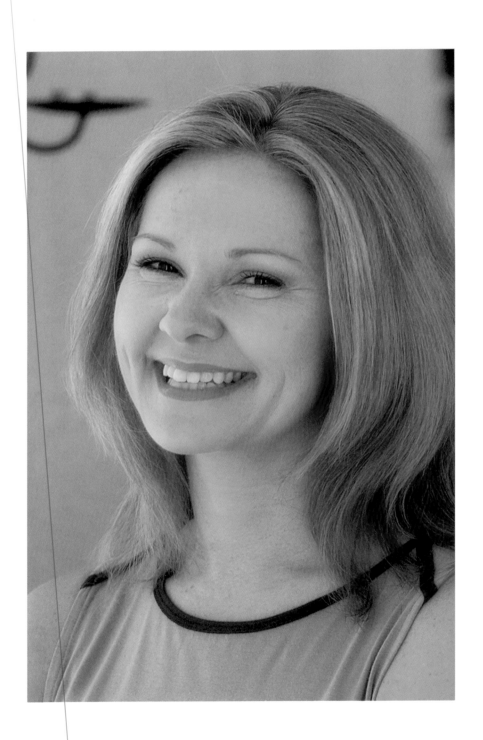

Introduction

My husband left this morning. I have asked him for a divorce, and he has agreed to a trial separation. I know in my heart this is over, that our relationship as we knew it has come to an end, but I am allowing him time to adjust and let go.

Separation is painful. It causes suffering. Patanjali, the mysterious author of the *Yoga Sutras*, knew this thousands of years ago. This work has been translated and is available to us today.[1] However, if we take a closer look inside, we know that we are never alone, that we are a part of a great, loving energy force that unites us all. That union is yoga, and it has helped me through many agonizing trials in this lifetime.

A broken heart takes many shapes. My divorce is not the first time or the last that I have known that pit of despair. In my own experience, I have felt loss not only through the termination of romantic relationships, but also through the death of loved ones, the end of friendships, betrayals, serious illnesses, abuse and addiction. It all amounts to a great deal of pain; but through the path of yoga, I have been able to pull myself through the many changes and transitions, from darkness into a lightness of being I never thought possible.

I am here to share these tools with you today. You may be in the midst of a world of hurt right now, but I assure you that underneath those layers of pain lies a deep well of true, honest-to-God joy. I have helped countless others in my yoga community who have walked through my studio doors, broken yet sceptical.

Finally, together we'll map out a sequence of yoga postures, from gentle warm-ups, to more active poses, exploratory movements, restorative poses, and a final meditation, so you may take this wisdom with you wherever you go.

CHAPTER I
My Story

When I was a little girl, I was a dreamer. I had giant expectations and believed everyone else felt the same way. I was a happy baby, had my basic needs met, didn't cry a whole lot, but soaked in everything. My father worked compulsively, my mother stayed at home to raise my little sister and myself. Dad drank, mom was an enabler; both were unhappy and unable to navigate their feelings. There was a lot of anger, sadness, and repression in my home growing up; and as I observed it all, gradually I became disappointed and emotionally shut down.

I spent a great deal of time alone, role-playing with my dolls, trying to block out the shouting in my surroundings. No wonder I have an affinity for turtles, with their ability to retreat into their shells. My father's drinking got worse, my mother's depression deepened, and I clung to my eclectic grandmother, who had a no-nonsense approach and who protected me with a fierce love.

When I was only four, I used to get up at 5:00 a.m. and do stretching with Jack La Lane, the fitness pioneer. I'd get out my orange and yellow daisy tea-party chair, and work to move the pain out of my little body. Sundays we would go to church, all dressed up for the Lord, and as I went through the ritualistic Catholic motions, I would stare at Jesus on the cross with a pleading eye, and speak directly to him, from the heart, asking him to please please please save me. And although I later gave up the Catholic faith, I learned from my mother and grandmother the path of deep devotion.

At age 13 it was time for confirmation, and I refused to go through the process. My family was horrified. I explained that I didn't want to be confirmed into a religion I wasn't sure was right for me – after all, I was still a kid. And to my amazement, our family priest agreed that I should be allowed to explore my faith before I took a life-long oath. So I set out to study world spiritual traditions, and what I discovered was that beneath all the differences, beneath the various perspectives and especially beneath the fighting were beautiful messages of love, honesty, non-violence, and peace that really resonated with me. I also discovered the ancient scriptures of yoga, which pre-dated most of these belief systems.

During this time, my family was in grave turmoil. Not as bad as some, but far worse than others. Dad was having affairs, mom was in deep denial, and I was becoming a teen. My hormones were all over the place. I tried to turn more to my studies, and became an A student, but that wasn't enough. I tried to be perfect, and kept coming up short in my parents' eyes. Like most of us at that age, I felt unworthy and awkward. As I grew breasts, I was ashamed of my sexuality, and my chest began caving in.

My father's drinking progressed into emotional and physical abuse, so I also turned to drinking and drugs. I went from the cheerleader girl-next-door to the party girl who could drink all the boys under the table, and I was proud of that! I smoked pot by age 14, drank a whole bottle of vodka the next year, and lost my virginity a couple of years later. I was looking for love, searching for something deeper; all this time I was reading the yoga scriptures but having no outside support.

At 16, my father finally lost it, and beat me so badly I left home. The reason? I was raped at a party, and he blamed it on me. I think I was more hurt and angry at my father than at the rapist. It was a scary time, and I moved from house to house until I graduated. I was suicidal and in a dangerous downward spiral. The turning point didn't come until I became an unwed mom in college.

Seems like an odd way to salvation, but I knew when I got pregnant I just had to knock it off – if not for myself, then for my unborn child. I longed to be a good mother, to bring her up with a respect and care that I had never known. I turned to therapy, traditional and alternative, and turned my life around.

One of the first steps on every spiritual path is looking at the truth. In yoga, truth is called *satya* in Sanskrit, and it is one of the first *yamas* or ethical guidelines in the Yoga Sutras, one of the oldest written documents on this path. Most people translate this as 'honesty toward others', which of course is an important value, but when directed toward ourselves it sheds a light that leads to all the other ethical truths, as well as the 'big' truth, that we are all one. There is no duality. We all hurt and we don't want to hurt.

Jesus said the truth shall set us free, and he was an enlightened guy. That doesn't mean it doesn't smart along the journey. In fact, usually this means a whole bunch of change, much discomfort, but is a needed step before the good stuff comes. It's kind of like getting your legs waxed. You know it's going to hurt a little, but it won't kill you, and in the end your legs will be silky smooth. Or, a less superficial example, you get a mammogram because in the end, getting your breasts cut off is a lot more painful than pressing them naked against a cold, hard plate.

In my case, it meant digging through all the little lies I told myself along the way, and learning to just 'sit with' the pain, witness it for what it was, forgive everyone involved, and learn the lesson. I had many lessons, many 'kicks in the butt' from the universe, before I started getting the bigger picture.

CHAPTER 2
What Happened:
Getting to the Truth

Remember your first break-up? I sure do. Felt like the world was coming to an end. Like someone was sitting on my chest. I actually went to the doctor once complaining of a 'heavy chest', and when all the test results came out normal, my physician just shrugged his shoulders.

My first real boyfriend broke up with me because I wouldn't kiss him in public. I remember wanting to, I was just flat-out scared and embarrassed. The next love of my life, after one starry night at a school dance, moved out of town. I spent the next five years thinking he was my missed opportunity, and we wrote many poetic love letters to each other. That is, until he came for a visit post-graduation and wasn't too keen on my new party-girl persona. He ended up making out with a close friend.

My first lover dumped me for someone else not too long after our 'first time'. Then the rape happened, and sex for me became a power play to get back at the male species, a way to be in control. I had a wonderful summer fling with a college student, who left me after I turned to Oreo cookies for solace; followed by another older man who I ended up living with when I was only 18, and who took care of me but was very volatile. The next year there was my daughter's father, who was nice on the eyes and who I knew a mere three months when I learned I was pregnant.

Post-birth, I took a solid year of finding myself before starting a string of failed relationships, each one starting with a huge high of endorphins, the intensity of infatuation, outrageous but emotionally cut-off sex, followed by the low of disillusion and disappointment. Again, I was looking for happiness outside of myself, for someone 'out there' to complete me, instead of already knowing I was perfect, divine even, exactly how I was. That realization is at the root of yoga, and would not come for me until much, much later.

In fact, it's a continual process of reminding myself of that inner glorious light we all share, when we're with someone, as well as when we are alone. In truth, we are never alone. We've probably heard this many times over, but as we grow on the spiritual path, as we evolve as a species, we must experience this at a deeper level. Often, this experience only comes after pain, turmoil, or a big fat wake-up call.

After news hits of your big loss, you are likely to feel shock, panic, denial, anger, grief, fear, you name it. Even if the loss comes because you have made the decision to change, any transformation carries a certain level of fear of what's to come. So the first step is to get to the truth of what happened – to 'sit with' the pain, unafraid to explore your emotions. You can make this happen even if you experienced the loss long ago and have not yet dealt with the pain. You must be honest about what happened before you can learn the lesson and progress, evolve, even shine.

Often I've found the best way to do this is to feel where we're manifesting the uncomfortable feelings in our body, and sometimes here, too, we may not know where to start. That's where the yoga poses come in. They are clues as to what's going on inside, starting at the physical realm.

Recently I attended a yoga workshop with a famous figure in western yoga circles. When we got to a hip-opening posture, pigeon pose, we held it for an extraordinarily long time. I've heard it said for years that our hips are the seat of our emotional drama, and they often hold just as much stress and tension, if not more, as the neck and shoulders. It's just easier to see the shoulders up near your ears when you are stressed out. My right hip in particular has given me trouble for some time, even real pain. I've had to back off from many a challenging pose because there was no room for it to move; it felt constricted and it just plain hurt.

But in this particular workshop, it must have been the right time and place to hear her words, the same directions I have given many times in leading my own class; and as I dropped into the sensation I began to cry. Not just any cry, but as Oprah says, the 'ugly cry'. I realized that I had been carrying this pain since I was first married, and not since childbirth, to which I had attributed its cause. And since pigeon pose lengthens all the deep, dense connective tissues in the hip rotators and the gluteus muscles, I realized this entire time my marriage was a literal 'pain in the butt', without me even recognizing it!

When I left that workshop, my pelvis felt free and light, and I've been pain-free ever since. I had seen doctors, chiropractors, acupuncturists, massage therapists, and no one had been able to release what that yoga teacher was able to facilitate in me that day. It was up to me to recognize when I was ready to let it go. When I decided to do so and gave my body permission to free up that particular pain, it just dissipated.

Just last night, as I was explaining a pose to a group of beginner yoga students, I reached around my back to bind my toe, expecting not to reach it because of the tight hips, when lo and behold, there it was – my toe in hand! Something even deeper had opened due to a combination of sustained, consistent practice, the acknowledgment and release of the emotional block in my body, and a willingness to suspend the thought that I could 'never' reach this pose.

The same could be said for transitioning in relationships. At first, we must face the pain, feel it, talk about it, negotiate the ending with our former partner, perhaps meditate on it, and listen for insights. This first step takes practice and patience, and can last a long time – or not, if the relationship was dead long before anyone acted on it. This part takes both effort and ease, as Patanjali also says in his Yoga Sutras. It takes determination to move through it, but also surrender – letting go of the end result. Ironically, when we are able to release control, we are often happily surprised.

The last step, meditation, is also important. Although I have been meditating for some time now, it is only recently I have committed myself to a half-hour sitting practice each morning. This has come about through a 12-step programme I have been following to help with my unfortunate addiction to chocolate chip cookies.

This morning, however, my sensory craving of choice wasn't sugar. In my quietest moments, now that I have taken food out of the equation, I am craving men. For months I have been churning over my marriage, and now I am entering a new phase of loneliness that I want to fill – it's a physical longing, like an itch that needs to be scratched. In my marriage, I filled the gap with food. Others may fill it with drugs, alcohol, shopping, gambling, even exercise. Mine was cookies. Not so bad, until the weight creeps on and you aren't so healthy any more.

In yoga, these sensory cravings are called *samskaras*, described best as grooves in the record of life. These grooves are patterns embedded deep in our psyche, habits formed over time but overcome as we create new, more positive grooves. How do we do this? Lots of will, support, patience, and a belief in something much larger than ourselves.

Often when I try to sit still, especially if I haven't released the restlessness through yoga postures first, my mind drifts off to these samskaras, going round in circles till I remember to listen to my breath. Other times, it wanders off to my lengthy to-do lists, my goals, my memories, my desires. Time and again I have to bring that monkey back to its tree, stop criticizing myself and trying desperately to escape like some kind of caged animal. When I've been able to sit within that circle of stillness, even if it's only for five minutes, the peace that comes is really indescribable.

That wasn't the case today. You see, last week I had my first real date in ten years. A wonderful man whom I met at my 20-year high-school reunion; someone I never gave the time of day to as a teenager, but is now consuming my thoughts and making my hormones go crazy. I know that I am a woman in transition, just mere months into a divorce, and that I should take longer to ease back into the dating world, but then there's that familiar gut ache of needing, of wanting to feel fulfilled and whole. It seems like this would be so easy to have with a romantic night at a local hotel.

I haven't succumbed yet, but only because I have been busy at my yoga studio and with my children. Thank God he has a daughter and work that keeps him occupied, too, so that we can't see each other, say, every minute. We have this chemistry that's intoxicating, despite the fact we know hardly anything about each other. My hope is that I can stop analyzing this attraction, to stay in the present and enjoy the moments we do share, without letting my mind (or my body) take over. Yoga teaches us first that we are not our bodies, although we need to take care of them and nurture them, and we are not our minds, not the chatter that fills our heads. We are indeed pure spirit, and that's my lesson learned today. It is that spirit that will fill me, guide me, make me whole – not a man, no matter how cute.

Along the path, we will meet many people who will lead us in the right direction, but we need to take the time to listen and pay attention. I have no doubt that I was meant to meet this new man in my life, and I prayed out loud in my car on the way to the reunion not for Mr Right, but for Mr Right Now. He is easy-going, gentle and affectionate, all ingredients I could use in my kitchen at the moment. Will we live happily ever after? Who knows? All I know is that I must be vibrating at a higher level to attract such an amazing person into my life, and if I don't make him the source of all my happiness and/or suffering, he could be someone with a message, a lesson to further me on my path to self-realization.

I have met many friends who wonder aloud constantly what they have done to deserve such poor treatment from their spouses, partners, significant others. If we observe all people as mirrors, we witness the truth that we attract people into our lives based on our own self-worth. If we feel we have nothing to offer, others will treat us as if we are nothing. Once we recognize our own brilliance, and have the courage to let that light truly shine, we will magnetically bring people to us who are like-minded and equally as loving.

I am no scientist; however, I once heard that we are made from the same gases and materials as all the stars in the sky. If you look out on a clear night and hold this idea, it can make you dizzy with awareness! It makes our problems seem small in comparison with the vastness of our universe.

When my mind won't behave, I visualize my belly filled with light, much like a shining star, and dwell within that brilliant centre. It balances me and gives me hope. Today, after a wrestling match with my ego mind, I brought my attention back to that centre of divine rays, and now I am feeling light and joyous.

I checked my phone messages – there's one from a student apologizing for sounding crazy, but wanting urgently to meet me with a message, a book to pass on. I am meeting her for lunch, and staying open for a chance at synchronistic opportunity. I am not thinking about my date tomorrow night.

CHAPTER 3
Denial into Truth

Mary came to my yoga studio through a mommy-and-me class. Her daughter and mine are very close in age, and they got along well together. In those early days, we didn't have many students, and those that came to mommy-and-me were usually the type who did lots for their kids, forgetting themselves in the process.

I thought this was the case with Mary, who walked in the door looking like someone had thrown a baseball into her chest. She is a beautiful woman who obviously takes good care of herself, but I had never seen anyone with such hunched shoulders at such a young age (my age, for goodness sake!).

Mary looked haunted. I wondered what her story was, but sensed I shouldn't pry. Besides, that's not my job as teacher. I facilitate the yoga, which may churn up a lot of memories and emotional baggage, but the processing part I leave to the students.

Surprisingly, Mary began crossing over from kids' classes to adult classes, regularly taking the gentle class, and gradually working her way up to more advanced classes. She asked me to help her through private sessions in her home, and we worked together closely for months. I gave her 'prescriptions', poses to practise on her own in between classes and our sessions, and unlike most of my clients, she was dedicated to her home practice and willingly did all I asked of her.

Her sleeping became sounder, and slowly she stood taller. In the beginning, when we would try triangle pose, I would work to lift her shoulder back, and she would wince and not budge. Now she was making real progress, due to her patience and motivation. It was such a pleasure to witness her growth and transformation, but I never asked her what happened to her to make her this way. She had been hurt deeply, that was obvious from her body language. Sure, her doctor made a formal diagnosis, but there was more to it than a simple malformation. Mary was protecting her heart.

Fast forward to the present, and Mary is now taking my yoga teacher training. While mentioning my divorce to her (I only tell a few select students my personal problems), she shared her story with me. Turns out she was married before, to a man who was clinically depressed and wouldn't help himself. When she finally got the courage to leave him, he committed suicide. Ah, the baseball to the heart...no wonder. But as she told me this, tears welled up in her eyes but didn't spill over. Instead, I saw a strength in her eyes I hadn't seen before. She had moved out of denial and into truth, into satya. And she is now well on her way to healing others.

CHAPTER 4
Agony into Acceptance

'*Come on in the light*
It feels right
Come on in the light
It's alright
Come on in the light
It's so right…
It's not a new song, it's a very old one.'
OLIVIA HICKS (FOUR YEARS OLD)

Last night I returned home after a long three-day yoga teacher training I'm in the middle of leading. It's an amazing experience, always refreshing to witness long-time students becoming teachers. Not only do we do lots and lots and lots of physical *asana* work, but we study *The Bhagavad Gita*[2] and the Yoga Sutras of Patanjali, and discuss our stories, our unique perspectives of how these ancient scripts affect our current state of affairs.

So I come home a little late due to traffic and an engaging post-training discussion, and my soon-to-be-ex is not happy about my tardiness. I try to apologize, but he is angry and storms out. My four-year-old daughter, Olivia, is obviously distressed by this interaction, and spends the rest of the evening crying for her daddy. This provokes a lot of guilt in me, as I hate to see my children suffer the consequences of my decisions.

It also hurts to hear her cry for her father, since I haven't seen her all weekend and miss her dearly. My ego wants her to cry for me, but I understand she is struggling to accept our separation, and it can't be easy for her to go back and forth between two houses that are so different. It's also awful to hear her anguish, but I listen as she keeps asking why, why, why, trying to acknowledge her pain and give answers appropriate to her level of development.

'Why are you and daddy divorcing? I don't like this. I want him to live here. He wants to come back – why won't you let him? I miss my daddy; I miss him; I miss him. Why?'

This is what I hear for hours. It is breaking my heart at a whole new angle. I want her to stop crying, to fix what's been broken, but I can't.

The truth is, she is on her own path and it is going to hurt for a long time, and all I can do is acknowledge that this must feel horrible for her and that I love her and always will. I just can't go back to her daddy. I just can't.

Before we can find insight and know peace, we must suffer and go through the pain of awakening. Satya is not easy sometimes. We are all like little kids, pleading for the answers, longing to fill the loss. As adults, sometimes we have to put aside our struggles for a time to nurture our children as they go through their own challenges.

If we can sit with their pain, hold it for them, perhaps they will learn how to do this for themselves. Somehow I was able to muster the strength to hold that pain for my child, even as her wails were deep down grating on my nerves. Imagine a world where we could all do this for our children.

We can face the truth of our life situations with the courage of a warrior. When we are able to face these painful truths and look them square in the eye without flinching, we can know peace. We will reach new levels of conscious awareness. As each individual learns these skills, very gradually we will reach a new dawning for our entire society, our world. The force that unites us within unites us all, and global transformation will come only as we learn this very personal process.

This morning is a new day. My daughter, now well rested, wrote her father a sweet letter in her mixed-up alphabet, attempting at a tender age to put to paper her feelings, much as I'm doing with this book. In the bathtub, she began singing the song that I've put at the beginning of this chapter. If that isn't transcendence, I'm not sure what is. This stuff works.

CHAPTER 5
Rage into Release

This morning, I am a menagerie of emotions. I have painful premenstrual cramps, despite my trip, yesterday, to the acupuncturist, who said I was stressed. My hormones are all over the place, raging against 'what I don't know'. I made myself go to the Farmer's Market yesterday after the acupuncture session, to collect healthy foods with my daughter. We even painted pottery – which should have been very therapeutic. On the way home, she may have been smiling, but I was simmering inside.

My ex-husband called to see if his text-messaging attempts had been successful. I wondered aloud why he just couldn't tell me what he had to say in person. I don't get the text-messaging craze, unlike my teenager. He wouldn't tell me, but with assistance I eventually got the messages. He was wondering if I could co-write a book with him called: How Yoga Saved my Marriage.

Very cute, I think. He's past the mean stage, where he's cursing me and basically behaving badly. Now we're on to wanting a reconciliation, without the apology. The pendulum swings, once again, in our divorce drama, and it just makes me downright mad.

Do I want to go to yoga right now? Hell no. I want to stay home and be pissed off. Thank God it's my job, and I have to go. But I know in my heart of hearts that this age-old science of yoga is the best way to transform my anger into a different kind of energy, a positive force for good, not evil. I need to move this stuff out of my body, before it mutates into worse cramps, or headaches, or some other malady.

I know this, but do I want to do it? No. I'm feeling like a small child right now, wanting to throw myself on the floor and refuse to go anywhere. My adult rational side, though, will get me into the shower and out the door.

This week has been great fodder for my book. I have not been able to write, which in addition to my yoga practice is my best release. My soon-to-be-ex-husband (there should be a name for this, like fiancé is to getting married) went on a huge drinking binge and tried to commit suicide. He ranted and raved, calling me 30 times in one day, and by the end of the week was in rehabilitation – thank the Lord. He is an alcoholic – and I had no idea how much he drank. That is the nature of the alcoholic, I guess, to hide things, and he was very good at this. And so I feel betrayed and very angry.

I took the week off from work, stayed with a good friend, cried and sat and hurt and talked and talked and vented and walked and did some gentle yoga and then did a very powerful yoga and now I am in this weird space of calm. Not sure if it's a peaceful calm, but I am in a numb stage, knowing intellectually that I need to take care of myself, to nurture myself in ways I know best, but not ready to move to forgiveness just yet. This will take time. I know this, but there is a lot of pain sitting under the surface of my calm, like lava in the volcano, and I would rather let that lava seep out than blow.

I thought for sure that my hip would act up in class yesterday, but it didn't. I should practise what I preach – no expectations. Instead, I had a flowing practice, followed by an engaging yoga teacher training with others on the path. This yoga is what saves me – as I breathe consciously, the chatter of my mind stills, and as I hold each pose, I stay present and centred, grounded in my body.

As I flow through *vinyasa*, my heart circulates and works tension out at a deeper level, and in the end, when I find the last savasana, I can lay in corpse pose with an empty mind and peaceful heart, able to face what comes up with an unshakable certainty. I surrender this all to God – Ishwara Pranidhara; another limb of the eight limbs of Ashtanga.

Never thought I'd be able to say that with a straight face, given my strict Catholic upbringing, but with all this yoga training and 12-step work, I know without a doubt that there is a higher power, a force that unites us all, and without it I just couldn't get by.

CHAPTER 6
Epiphany: Learning the Lessons

Of course, yoga class went great. By the next day, however, I learned it was not premenstrual syndrome (PMS) cramps as I had thought, but an intestinal flu that's been going around. Shows what I know. I had prayed for help in losing my last ten pounds, and even though I've heard that's quite a common prayer, no matter what our size, God said, 'Well OK.' I should have been more specific. Be careful what you wish for, 'cos it might just come true.

During my few days on the sidelines, I was faced with yet another conflict – another opportunity to transform anger. This time the answers came through rest and meditation instead of movement. While ill, I was faced with trying to figure out what I could eat that wouldn't pass right through me.

I was feeling weak and knew I needed sustenance, but wasn't sure what could work that would also fit into my eating plan. My food sponsor kept insisting I have a plan, but I kept insisting that I eat what my body needs to get back into balance. If that meant a little more rice and less salad for now, so be it. I figured I'd get support; instead I received judgement.

This was disappointing, to say the least. My first response was to try to call a friend and talk it out, but it was too early in the morning to call anyone. I also wanted to go for a walk or do some yoga poses, but I was still too weak and achy to get out of bed. So I sat with it, and the answer came pretty darn quickly. This programme was just too much: too much structure, too much pressure to be perfect, too much judgement. Despite the founders' good intentions, I think any time humans try to regulate our lives to an extreme, it creates separateness. Separateness creates suffering, and I was indeed suffering.

Yet I am afraid of failing. I have lost weight through this programme, and feel healthier than I've ever felt in my life. I'm not sure I can keep it up on my own. But in my quiet moments, I know I need to try. I found another similar 12-step programme that seems a little gentler, a little more forgiving. And the meetings fit my schedule better – perhaps that's a sign.

Last week, I had a vivid dream that I was visiting Oprah, and I went to her personal bakery and started gorging myself on pastries. Oprah came over to me and put her arms around my shoulders, just saying, 'It's all right, we do the best we can.' My fears were coming out in my subconscious mind, and Oprah, who has always been a mother figure to me, came to nurture me in my dreams.

Movement can indeed work emotions out of the body, when the body is in a healthy state to do so. The trick is learning to tap into what's right for your body, to use your intuition and guidance from a higher power, and follow through with that guidance. Sometimes it's best to rest, and if anyone tells you not to follow your gut feeling, often it's better to go your own way.

I have been feeling lost this last week. Again, unable to write, stuck in my longing for fulfilment, for peace of mind, for chocolate, for sex, for good wine. Sometimes, the further I travel on this path, the more it circles back to the beginning, much like an elaborate labyrinth. Once, my friend Jennifer, my eldest daughter, then only ten-ish, and I set out on a hike to the Berkeley Hills to find a set of man-made labyrinths we'd heard about.

We found a giant one first, and as we slowly walked to the centre, representing the centre of our own heart that many have travelled, we found a quirky altar of sorts. Those who had been here before us had placed pictures, poems, trinkets and various memorabilia on this altar. We had brought nothing, but decided to make wishes anyway. As we closed our eyes and did so, the wind picked up and gave us all chills – from the inside out. I had wished for truth, Jennifer for love, and my daughter wouldn't tell us what she wished for. It was left a mystery (like the other alleged labyrinths we never found). Apparently, it was the magical ingredient.

Again, be careful what you wish for, because the very next day we all had some major truths open up in our respective love lives. Some were unexpected twists of fate. I was able to find closure in an old relationship – he showed up on my front doorstep! Not sure what happened with my daughter, but I know that she was able to open up more after that day, to find love at a new familial level.

Last night, I felt a similar natural phenomena leading me to the conclusion that all my longings, all my little problems are just plain insignificant. After co-teaching a beginners' yoga class with one of my interns, deep into *savasana* corpse pose at the end we all felt and heard a giant bang, like someone ran a car into the studio, followed by a rumbling below us – an earthquake!

I had asked my higher power to give me a sign, some direction to follow, something so that I could surrender and leave this uneasiness to the flow of the universe. And boom! I got a big bang and a gentle shaking – no damage, just a little reminder of the power and glory of spirit, of mother nature, of God, Buddha, Krishna – whatever name this force takes. Doesn't matter, we were all awed.

Now I know others felt the earthquake, too. I learned later it was four point something on the Richter scale, and based in Glen Ellen, not too far from us. But in savasana, on the ground, post-yoga practice, it was particularly poignant. One student, who recently finished her bar exam and had lost a former spouse to cancer, told me the earthquake was exactly what she needed to remember how small we all really all. That isn't to say we are insignificant, but our problems sure are. This life as we know it could all be gone in a flash of glory, and we need to live live live, to connect, to dance, to see the light in each other's eyes, and just plain surrender the small stuff. Can you do this today?

Whenever my birthday rolls around, I get super reflective. Another year lived, and what am I going to do next? This year, due to all the transformation around me, especially the break-up of my marriage, I decided to do something to mark the occasion. I essentially have all the material 'things' I need, outside of paying off all my bills and maybe a yacht, so I am working to gather experiences, and in the process, maybe face my fears and learn a few lessons.

I have wanted to get a tattoo for a while now, but there was that nasty fear of needles getting in the way. I already have one of a turtle on my right shoulder blade that I got in Hawaii, after a week of relaxing and seeing lots of 'normal' people with them, not just the sailors and whores my mom said had them. The turtle was surprisingly not that painful, but I never thought I'd be the type to want another. I guess it's true what they say: they are addictive. I also suppose you could consider it an adornment of the body, but for me it was symbolic of my new-found independence.

Fortunately, a new tattoo 'salon' opened up down the street from my yoga studio recently, and when I met the artist I knew it was another 'sign' to move forward with my plans. His salon looked more like a day spa than a tattoo parlor, which eased my fears and phobias right away, and he had a very laid-back way about him. I brought in some images off the Internet for him to combine into a lower-back tattoo, sexy yes, but also on my root chakra region, an area connected to family of origin.

I was delighted with his sketch of a lotus flower, a symbol that means a lot of things to different people/spiritual traditions, but for me represents rising out of the mud, new growth, and non-attachment (the dew drops just roll off the petals). Above the flower is an 'om' symbol, considered universal sound, the spiritual noise at the centre of our universe. Green vines are growing out from the blossom, symbolizing the spiritual seeds I hope to plant with my yoga studio, with little hearts along the vines spreading love.

So you can see I was pretty psyched up about this endeavour, especially after I went ahead and plopped down the deposit money and made the appointment. But when I arrived with my girlfriends beside me, after an hour of prep work – shaving my back, cleaning it with alcohol, applying the stencil – I was absolutely terrified.

I tried using my breath work, my girlfriends even breathing with me audibly, but nothing was working. I was sick to my stomach, light-headed and feeling quite faint. This was before the needles – or points, as Auric called them. We had King Kong playing on the video-cassette recorder (VCR); I even gave in and took a tranquilliser, which only served to make me groggy.

So by the time the needle dug in, I just couldn't handle the pain. Every time he applied the tip, my muscles involuntarily contracted, and all that wincing was making the artist's work turn into scribbles. After one little squiggle, I cried mercy. I just couldn't do it. Now I had a $50 squiggle permanently etched on my rear. I went back to my friend's house filled with disappointment and napped for a few hours.

The next day, when all my students began asking about the new tattoo I had bragged about the week prior, I had to tell them the truth. I said the squiggle was Sanskrit for 'coward'. It was, after all, a little funny.

I believe that things do happen for a reason, and I planned to sit with this and figure out why I chickened out, why it seemed so fortuitous for the tattoo place to open up when it did, only for me to bow out. I dedicated my Saturday practice to this mystery, and then was able to let it go.

Later in the day, I had a Thai massage, where you are tugged and pulled into different passive yoga postures. He reminded me that the lower back is a place where people tend to carry their anger issues. I also realized during the massage how tight my jaw was feeling, that I must be grinding my teeth a lot, which you normally do when you are angry or resentful.

And then it dawned on me. I was still angry about this divorce: angry at my former spouse for his lies, his alcoholism, his betrayal of my trust. It brought all my anger issues from childhood, from trusting my daddy as only a child could and his own inability to face his feelings and fears, using the alcohol as a crutch, a cover-up.

Of course I'm still angry! Who wouldn't be? But being me, I tend to get impatient and want those 'bad' feelings to disappear at once. I was numb, not over it, and my body was telling me loud and clear that I needed to face this stuff first before I can move on and get to the 'good' stuff. My squiggle now symbolizes this process for me, and I am glad for it. It's now my mark of courage.

So now what, goshdarnit. Well, I am writing. I went for a walk this morning, that's a good start. I repeated a mantra, Rama, suggested by Eknath Easwaran, the prolific scholar whose translation of *The Bhagavad Gita* I read each morning. 'Ramaramaramarama', I say to myself as my faithful dog trots along beside me, and I am on the verge of tears.

Yes, this stinks; I am so very pissed. I admit it. It is my day off from yoga, and my body needs a good rest, so I will not do any physical poses today. But I can acknowledge that the pain is there, and ask God, Jesus the Christ, Buddha the compassionate one, Allah, whomever, to take this anguish away. I get on my knees and pray, in a very direct, begging sort of way, to let this anger fly out of my body; to let me trust like a child again, to regain that lost innocence.

'I've learned the lesson, Lord,' I say out loud.

We'll see how it works out.

OK, so maybe I have a helluva lot to learn. This weekend, wrapped up in my ego-world of pain and hurt after such profound revelations, I managed to mess things up with my girlfriend, the one who opened up her house to me when my ex was acting scary, who breathed with me when my tattoo was hurting and has never judged me once, who has been nothing but loving and supportive when so many others have not.

We went out, and without getting into embarrassing details, I ended up betraying her trust, hurting her deeply, and regretting my actions. I have behaved very badly this weekend. I was feeling like I couldn't trust others, so I somehow managed to hurt the one person who trusted me completely.

So today I feel guilty, dirty, shameful, empty. My heart is feeling more broken than ever; it really feels like an open wound. Can't understand how after such profound discoveries into my psyche, my soul, I could be so selfish. Guess I'm human after all. It may be a while before my meditation takes me to *nirvana*; maybe a few more lifetimes. Oh well, something else to sit with today.

It is overcast and cold, despite being August, and the weather matches my mood. The reunion guy finally called this morning, cancelling our weekend plans, again, and stating that he really isn't blowing me off. I don't know what to believe or who to trust. I am at the end of my rope. I am lonely, I am sad. I am going to go meditate now.

CHAPTER 7
Negotiation: Acknowledging the Agreements

We can learn a lot from our kids. They are much smarter than us – no baggage. We start out so pure, so innocent, so trusting … then we get wounded. I was asking a friend, who just happens to be a therapist, for advice the other night. How do I start trusting again? How – when my father, my former boyfriends, my ex-husband – have all lied to me, betrayed my trust again and again, how can I learn to trust others and stay open, to find intimacy and true love?

She told me to look to my daughter, who is only four. She still trusts me completely. This is our agreement: I take care of her needs, and she just loves me unconditionally. So yesterday, when I was feeling sad and sorry for myself, I took her out to a teddy-bear factory, and we made each other stuffed animals with our voices inside, with messages of love. Of course, the outing didn't quite fit my initial expectations.

She started sobbing in line because she wanted to make one for her father, too, and I didn't have enough money for all of us. In hindsight, I should have just let her make one for her dad instead, but my birthday is this week and I wanted a damn bear for myself to hug. So she cried throughout the store, and we didn't get to make the birth certificates. The clerks tried to console her to no avail, and I didn't explain, just said she felt like crying, I guess.

We went for ice cream and she stopped crying when we dressed our bears – hers in heart pyjamas, mine in belly-dancing gear. We carried those bears around all day, nurturing them, hugging them, getting plenty of smiles from other passers-by not used to seeing a grown woman dragging around a belly-dancing brown bear. But in that nurturing, she found her solace, and in loving her and being present to her needs, I helped heal myself.

Once, a few months back, my Olivia was practicing yoga on her own, creating new poses. I asked her what yoga pose she was doing, and she looked straight in my eye and said it wasn't a pose. She was practising love; 'I practise it every day,' she said.

We can choose every day to practise love with whomever we share a relationship, not just romantic ones. We can practise love just by smiling with whoever we come in contact with. This, too, is yoga.

Problem is, when we enter into romantic relationships, we are loaded with expectations as to how this person should act, should be, and when they don't fit our image of perfection, we practise judgement, not love. We are disappointed, let down. In the beginning, we are just high on endorphins. We don't really know much about this person at all except we are attracted to their physical body and we want them to like us back. We flirt, we toy around, we have fun together, but when a few months roll around (three–six to be exact) our true natures tend to surface, and we enter into certain agreements, usually without any sort of awareness of what we are agreeing to.

For instance, filled with love for my daughter this morning, after a night of hugging our bears and each other, I awoke late to the reunion guy's phone call. I missed the call, but his message was another little heartbreak – he was cancelling our date again after not seeing him for five weeks. Thank goodness I knew enough to make the date the day after my birthday to avoid disappointment, but it was still sad. He gave all the right excuses: his mother was in town, his daughter was going back to school soon, and the following week he had free, maybe we could get together then?

A light went on for me this morning. His excuses may be all legitimate, but I need to love myself more and set up a boundary here. Enough is enough. I was disappointed enough in my marriage, why would I wait around when I'm just dating? He is who he is, and I'm not going to change him, but hey, this ain't working. If he were really that into me, he'd find a way to see me.

Unconsciously, we had already set up an agreement. He would see me, on his terms, when he had the time, and when that time came I would reorganize my life to meet his needs.

I am so not going to do this any more. All it takes to change this pattern is awareness, and my vision just got a lot clearer today. Yes, I will trust, I will accept, I will love, but I won't be waiting in the wings. I just can't any more.

People energetically get what they put out. We are all vibrating on different levels, different wavelengths. That much is scientific. I have been putting it out there that I am a lap dog, waiting under the table for whatever scraps of attention and affection I can get. When I know deep down that I deserve more, I will attract someone who can give more. This I know is true, but it takes more practice, more sitting, more reflecting, more love.

I think I am finally ready today to negotiate a real honest-to-God legal agreement: my parenting plan. Not sure if my ex will agree to it or not, but I'm ready to put it on paper for me, without resentment, without anger, without grief. And someday I'll be ready to put onto paper what I am looking for in a mate, but not now. I'm not really sure yet. I can't trust my wounded nature. I need to work on being whole, first.

Once I am whole, filled with a higher divine love, and I'm able to see once more the love of God shining through everyone's eyes, I won't have to look so hard for a love match. It will happen when I'm ready, when I trust not in another, but in the love of the Lord, in the positive ebb and flow of the universe.

CHAPTER 8
Peace: a Path

Today I am lunching with my father for his birthday. We are all born within a few weeks of each other in my family of origin – a pack of Leos, all fighting to be the centre of attention. Small wonder we share so much drama. This morning I called him, despite the fact that we rarely talk, and wished him well. I let him talk and I just tried to listen as he complained about the swimming pool he now says he wishes he could bulldoze.

That swimming pool is a symbol of real pain for me, because once upon a time he said he couldn't afford to send me to college, and then turned around and got a loan for that big, below-ground pool. It was a slap in the face to me, but was also the impetus for real independence; I knew if I really wanted to make college happen, it was up to me, not my family.

I went through a lot of heartache, even clinical depression, but eventually I came through to the other side. My dad is who he is. He's pretty selfish, but aren't we all? I still graduated from college, with high marks, because I was determined. And I did it all by myself; something I'm very proud of.

So today as he was ranting at the pool for having to clean and patch it up, I wanted to say something about karma biting him in the ass, but I didn't. I just listened. He is who he is. I don't have to like him, don't have to be his friend, but he did bring me into the world and I can listen to his pain without judgment and wish him a happy birthday.

It is these types of decisions, made on a daily, even moment-to-moment basis, that create peace. We choose whether or not to create drama, whether to escalate an argument, whether to push our opinion on others in an effort to prove we are right. Ultimately, what is the price of being right all the time? It's exhausting. Of course, when others are trampling all over your rights, you have the right to set up a boundary, to calmly state your case, and when necessary, to walk away. That part I'm still learning.

It's a fine, fine line we walk, learning how to get along with others. But I wouldn't trade it for the world. In the ancient yogic scriptures, it is how we get to *samadhi*, to *nirvana*. We could sit under a tree for a million years and wait for enlightenment to come, we could travel to the Himalayas and hide out in a cave and practise levitation and such. Or we can choose to practise love, to practise serving others while loving ourselves completely, with devotion, with faith. It is a choice, and choices give us power. It is this power, not the kind of power that works to destroy others, that brings lasting peace.

When we bring peace into our lives on the small scale, this peace ripples out to help the world. We must do our part. It seems small, but it is the hardest thing. Next time you are faced with a conflict, how will you react? You may feel the anger, that is normal and human, but what will you do with that anger? You could rage against the person you blame for your anger, either yourself or someone else. You could get violent, in words and/or action. You could turn that anger inward and manifest disease. Or you could calmly state your case and let it go. Walk away. Walk away; and when that anger still infects your body, do some yoga asanas. It helps.

One of my yoga teachers asked me how I could have lunch with my father on his birthday, after all that he did to me. He wondered what I 'needed to get out of it'. The truth is, after many years of searching, I have no emotional charge around him any more. He is my father, and he brought me into this world, and he is very wounded, as we all are.

I see him now, as an adult, through eyes of compassion, and I have forgiven him long ago. I forgave him, not because I forgot what he did to me, not that I 'let him off the hook', but because the hatred would have become a parasite and taken me over, body and soul. I knew I had to get rid of that poison, or it would destroy me, not him.

My father is already in his own hell, a hell of his creation. He has his own demons to contend with: a cold mother, a passive father, both who passed away without any closure in their relationships. As a child, I was not in a position to forgive him, for he had all the power; but as an adult, I have the power: the power to choose to accept him for who he is, not how I wish he would be.

Will he ever say he's sorry? No way. Will he ever be the daddy I longed for growing up, who would sweep me into his arms and make me feel safe, loved, protected? No. But I can do that for myself. It takes work, hard work, but I can love myself the way I want my father to love me. He can't even love himself unconditionally, how is he supposed to love anyone else that way? I believe I chose him as my parent in this lifetime, to teach me the lessons I need to learn to grow on my path. It's up to me to take those lessons to heart.

Peace is basically three steps: truth/acceptance, compassion/ forgiveness, unconditional love. You can use these steps in every relationship, every conflict, every situation. They have been taught by all the masters throughout history, from Jesus to Buddha to Krishna.

In yoga class, students usually come to class initially because they wish either to lose weight or to heal the body from some injury or illness. They may have some awareness that yoga helps ease stress, and everyone is all stressed out these days, so they figure they could use help in that area, too. After trying out a practice session, either they feel really fantastic and are not really sure why, or certain things come up for them from the emotional body that they aren't ready to face yet and they make excuses that's it's too hard, too easy, too expensive, they are just too busy, and they don't return.

Every person is on their path, and I try hard not to take it personally when people don't come back. As a new teacher, I used to feel like it was all my fault, that I didn't teach a good enough class, that I wasn't a good enough teacher. But the truth is, some people will like the class, others won't. For some, all those excuses will get in the way. For others, those excuses are there for now, and perhaps someday in the future, some trigger, some loss, will help them come back to their practice, either through me, or some other spiritual path.

But in the beginning it's all about the body. Yoga, done consistently, will indeed create a healthy, toned body. I could go into all the benefits and detail them out pose by pose. That alone will make you feel good, will give you energy. But what happens after the body is healthy and toned, when it is free of illness and pain? Then what will your inner judge talk about? If you are no longer too fat or too thin, too sick, or too victimized by the world, then what? Once our bodies, our temples are fit, we notice what's going on in our minds, and that's where we can start to face the truth.

Every single day I get phone calls from mostly women asking if they do yoga will they get a better body, will they lose that last ten pounds? The truth is, if you came to class every day for a week, you would lose weight, but would you be happy? Would it be enough?

Many women tell me they are just too fat to do yoga, so in my mind I start thinking of ways to help modify the poses to accommodate a larger physique, and when they come in through the door, they are most often of average size. Sure, they may have put on some pounds as they worked too hard, took care of their kids and ate their leftovers, stopped by too many a fast-food place. But in their heads, compared to their younger selves or their idealized image of what they should look like, they are enormous.

So the first step is taking an honest-to-God assessment. When I had my younger daughter, I was on doctor-ordered bed rest for most of my pregnancy (six months) and gained 60 pounds. Plus, all my muscles atrophied without any movement, so I was like a giant blob. While I was thrilled to have a happy, healthy baby, I couldn't look at myself in a mirror, or even my reflection in store windows as I walked by. There was a lot of self-loathing going on inside as I didn't recognize my body any more.

But I bought some larger yoga clothes, and had to humbly start my practice over again, adjusting for my new size. In all the twisting poses, my bigger tummy would get in the way, but I kept reminding myself that with each twist, I was helping aid my digestion, which would ultimately whittle that waist down again. I worked to see myself as my baby daughter did: perfect, whole, and complete.

During this time I took a job teaching yoga part-time at a gym. I went to my first staff meeting not knowing any of the instructors, and overheard a conversation between them about how fat they were. These women pretty much epitomized the womanly ideal of perfect bodies, yet still they weren't satisfied.

They worked out for hours and hours, every single day, obsessed over their perceived imperfections and deprived themselves of any food deemed the least bit unhealthy. Truth is, it's not perfection we are seeking, but acceptance and self-love. And we only get that self-love through practice, through letting ourselves 'off the hook', and through complete forgiveness.

If you commit to practising a realistic amount of times per week, you can begin to let go of that need to be perfectly thin, perfectly fit. If you are practicing steadily, you are doing the best you can and your body will respond within its own limits. Hopefully your studio or the place where you practise will be free of mirrors. Students often complain in the beginning that they can't see if they're doing a pose 'right' because I have no mirrors in my studio.

But the truth is, if there were mirrors they still wouldn't be able to see, from a one-dimensional perspective, if they have correct alignment. They would be too busy judging what they look like in their reflection. The mental chatter would be going full throttle, and their minds would be comparing their bodies with other bodies, for better or worse, competing to be the best. Imagine the conversation; you've probably had a similar one in your own head:

'Look at that pimple on my chin. I should have worn make-up today to cover it up. Why am I still getting zits at my age? Look at the way my fat falls over my pants – ooh, yuck. That chick next to me looks like she's in pain. At least I look better than her, and I have no idea what I'm doing. Wish I had that woman's boobs …'.

Instead of keeping a calm inner centre, suddenly we're thrust into an inner dialogue that is just plain crazy. The mind will do this, to move about like a monkey (as the Buddhists call it) or like an untrained puppy dog. It is up to us to be the alpha dog and bring the mind back to the present, using our breath, listening to the sounds of our life force moving through us.

The instructor is there to help adjust the student so they are moving physically in the right direction, reminding us that when it hurts we've gone too far, to listen to our bodies' messages carefully instead of being distracted by the inner critic. In this way, we learn. Our bodies make a mental imprint of what the pose should feel like, so the next time we enter the posture, our body remembers and responds.

So we face the truth: We have come to this place in our bodies through living our busy lives, through the choices we've made, and we take responsibility and ownership of those choices. They are not right or wrong, they are just the choices we made based on the information we had at the time. We ate too much when we were stressed, or were celebrating, vacationing, poverty stricken, whatever. We didn't have time to exercise because we were way too busy, too tired, too fat.

Bottom line is, we're ready to get healthy, to feel better about the choices we make moving forward. We only have to choose to be right here, right now, practising health through meditation and motion.

Next comes forgiveness. We may feel guilty, shameful for the choices we have made. We over-indulged on that last cruise, we ate at McDonald's three times last week and ate pizza the other four. We have been paying dues at the health club for four years and have only gone five times.

It is what it is. Forget all the little lies you've told yourself about why you can't be healthy and happy, the lies about how ugly and terrible and pathetic you are. Forget the lies others tell you, the broken promises, the manipulations, for they are only coming from their own wounded natures. You are a divine child of God, perfect in every single way. Get that? You are perfect! Don't hide from it; let it shine. That is true power, and you already have it in you, every second of every day.

Remember the end of the Wizard of Oz? Dorothy and her friends went through all of those trials and tribulations, through evil forests and wicked witch treatment, only to find that she had the power to go home all along.

You, too, have your own ruby slippers. Sometimes you just forget they're there. You take your shoes for granted, even though they are a spectacular shade of red. If you remind yourself daily that those ruby slippers are there, that they are spectacular, sooner or later you'll believe it and own your power. You'll also see that power shining out of the eyes of others, and remember that we all have it. You'll find compassion for others, but first you must find it for yourself.

When you've discovered the ease of forgiveness, that it really is just a choice to not beat yourself up any more, the love comes organically. Love will heal all the pain you've ever suffered – but you have to practise it, too.

Yesterday was a big day for me. My reunion guy gave me yet another excuse why he couldn't make it out to see me this weekend, that he needed to cancel our plans post-birthday because his mother was in town – again. He cancelled his work to see her, even though he had said he couldn't cancel his work for me.

In the middle of our phone conversation, I got a call on the other line from my eye doctor to confirm an appointment. They wanted me to call them back to confirm, rather than just leave a message. Interesting. That call was a message to me from God: time to see this dating situation clearly with my eyes wide open.

After listening carefully to his excuses, I told him the truth. I felt disappointed, and that it seemed that this just wasn't working. I was disappointed often in my marriage, and I didn't wish to be disappointed when I was dating. I told him this isn't his fault or mine, it just wasn't going to work out. The truth is, we haven't seen each other in five weeks, and logistically it was just too difficult to work out.

Of course, he tried to give more excuses, and tried to open it up for the following week when his daughter was away, but something shifted in me and recognized that this was over. I wasn't going to rearrange my whole schedule to meet his. If he really wanted to be with me badly enough, he'd find a way.

So this made me sad, and I went to work to teach a yoga class, and of course it made me feel better. My girlfriend came over after class and we cried together as she said she forgave me for my betrayal and she loved me and wanted me in her life. On the way home, buoyed up by her capacity to forgive and love, I pretended that I was in love, infatuated with life and its wonders. I have been infatuated a few times in my life now, and I can bring back to mind those intoxicating, heady feelings at will. How you don't feel hungry at all, that the sunsets seem more colourful, people around you seem to smile more brightly.

Why not practise that feeling – any time? When we are in the first stages of love, most of those feelings are created when the other person isn't even around physically, so why can't we bring those feelings to the forefront through the power of our will? The truth is, we can. I did it yesterday, and I feel like Scrooge on Christmas day after his visit from the three spirits of past, future, and present.

Transformation is available whenever we choose, right here, right now. Why don't you try it for yourself?

CHAPTER 9
Allowing for Answers

Tonight is my birthday eve. My birthday celebrations usually last about a week. And since the tattoo idea didn't work out exactly as planned, I went to a psychic with my aforementioned friend with the amazing capacity to forgive. We drove an hour and a half through the country, not sure what the heck we were doing and not sure if we should spend the money, but felt compelled to do so anyway, for some answers.

Well, it was indeed worth the money. I got my answers. In a nutshell, the reunion guy was just a lesson, not a life partner (I knew it); I needed to get away to the beach to heal and let my new teacher trainees fly solo, even if they're still green. I need to file my damn divorce papers once and for all, and when I do, all kinds of wonderful stuff is going to happen. If I stay on this spiritual path, I will meet my soul mate in four–five months, but if I don't 'do the work', if I don't own my power and face the conflict, the mess of my divorce, I will put off my soul mate for another year or longer, and he won't be happy.

This all rings true to me, and tonight's yoga class made my heart sing. I felt like crying, and I never cry when I teach yoga, only when I am the student. In bridge pose, my heart opened three sizes, like the Grinch after he learned his lesson. I saw a bright green colour radiating from my chest, and blue, too, in my throat chakra, the chakra of truth and self-expression. I have never had my heart feel that open before, that expanded, and it felt great, really great.

I came home to a project my ex-husband was working on: a vegetable garden plot in our backyard. He was so proud, and then so disappointed when I didn't hug him, just told him a sincere thank you. I know he wants more, and he is just going to hang on for dear life to our marriage, which in my mind has been dead in the water for some time. I feel compassion for him, I do, but that is all. It is over, and I need to deal with the mess, to move forward. There is going to be no easy way out of it, and I have been putting it off for weeks now.

The psychic said it's easier to move through hell when you know heaven, your bliss, is on the other side. I feel she is right, on a deep cellular level, and all is good. Happy birthday to me.

My lessons are coming fast and furious. I am being tested, that I know for sure. The last few weeks have been a tsunami of emotion, and I am the surfer riding the crazy waves. I can do this. I read a verse from *The Bhagavad Gita* early this morning – really early, couldn't sleep – like I try to do each morning. Easwaran's insights truly hit home for me, and this morning in particular, the poignancy of the verse made my eyes fill with tears:

'Who serves both friend and foe with equal love, not buoyed up by praise or cast down by blame, alike in heat and cold, pleasure and pain, free from selfish attachments and self-will, ever full, in harmony everywhere, firm in faith – such a one is dear to me.'[3]

Easwaran draws from the lives of mystics and saints, of Gandhi and St Teresa of Avila, to demonstrate how the power of love may transform, to show how it is possible – in fact, I believe it is the real goal of life – to love our opponents, our enemies the same way we love our friends. And nowhere does this seem more necessary than in the battlegrounds of divorce.

I met with my ex-husband's rehab counsellor the other day. He was supposed to meet us for a kind of mediation, but he didn't show. That was probably a good thing, as I was a bit unnerved, knowing I would need to set some boundaries and speak my truth, and not sure I would have the same courage to do this in front of him, as we have old patterns, like most couples.

The opportunity to speak with the counsellor first was a blessing, and judging from the books on her desk, she is on her own spiritual path. We had a common ground, and she shared that she, too, had been in an unhappy marriage with an alcoholic for many years. I told her what was going on, from my perspective, of course, and we set a new appointment for a few days later, this time letting the ex know he really needed to be there for some healing and closure.

I think he believed he was there to prove his love for me, to get me back, to show what a changed man he'd become. We started the session with him affirming how the rehabilitation programme and the 12 steps have transformed him, and as he spoke I could feel myself tense up, to want to say, '…. yeah, but …' only I refrained. I let him talk, trying to hold some compassion for this man I was married to for eight years, who like me, has probably been through hell these last few months and, like me, is trying to make some sense out of his life.

The difference being, he is just really waking up now that the fog of alcohol is gone, and now the real work begins. He has no idea what he's up against, when the deep pain hits – like it does for us all. Will he have the strength to not cover his emotions with alcohol, food, sex, whatever? I've been doing this for decades now, and it's still difficult, but it does get easier.

So I'm having compassion for him, and when it was time for me to talk, I spoke my truth, clearly, calmly, detached, but from my heart. He fidgeted in his chair, and wanted to interrupt, but couldn't with the third party present. I was in a safe place, and I was able to find the courage to acknowledge what I heard from him, but also say it just wasn't what I wanted in my life right now, that I was ready to move forward without him; and he was going to have to accept this and move on.

I know this must have hurt him deeply, but the counsellor was there to reflect my words and help him pick up the pieces. I'm not yet sure if he really 'got' all I said, for later he called late at night with a dead tone in his voice, saying I was killing him, that no one would ever love me like he did. I told him to reach out to his sponsor, that I needed to take care of me right now.

Before, his words would have stung. Now I know he's wrong: no one can ever love me like I can love me, like the universe can love me, for I am a part of that divinity and his words are controlling and hurtful, not loving. I must love me, must feel whole and complete with this deep love, and then nothing, no one, can hurt me. Wow. This I know is true.

So yes, this process, which could continue for years, is both painful and empowering. I can face him like a warrior, but a peaceful warrior. I will not tear him down, but I will tell the truth. I take responsibility for not telling this truth during our ten years together, but I do not regret that path, for it has taken me to this place of unity.

And after that painful encounter, I returned to the man I met just last week, whom I locked eyes with at an outdoor concert on a warm August night under the stars, whom I feel like I've known for ever, that we just picked up where we left off ... We can't stop talking and sharing, and his kisses make me want to sob somewhere deep. Is this the soul mate the psychic spoke of? Is her timing off, for it's too soon. I asked her this, and she says anything is possible. Anything is possible.

Her timing on other predictions has been off for me in the past. And Lord knows, I am doing the work. But I promise not to analyze this one. I am speaking consciously within the inner recesses of my mind when we're together ... be present, be present, be present. It is my latest mantra. My heart is racing like a teenager in infatuation, but this is different and new. And this time, I am open and aware, in love with the divine connection in the universe, plugged in, knowing that it is OK to be fearless in loving, no matter where it takes me. I can't imagine ever marrying again, but I am not afraid to love and get hurt any more because I know I'll survive. I can risk this, I can.

And of course, like attracts like. He separated from his wife the same month as me – we are at the same place. We can help each other get through the pain of our respective divorces, as long as we can stay out of blame and resentment for our ex-partners – for our own sakes, as well as our children (he has two girls, too). So no matter what happens with this relationship, we are here right now to further each other on our path, and I am happy: happy happy happy.

I smashed my left middle toes in a weird accident yesterday, and I am still happy. In pleasure and in pain I am happy, for I am free in the knowledge that everything happens for a reason, that now I can take some time off to sit and meditate and work on this book, to put some closure on my divorce, and hang out with my new 'partner', to be with my kids and love them fiercely through all this transformation and show them how to be strong in the face of opposition, to be loving in the midst of chaos.

So I admit, it's been tough to write about heartbreak when the last few weeks I've been giddy in infatuation. Fortunately, I believe it's much more than that. I have a real connection with this guy, and we've been pretty inseparable lately. Thank God for whatever it is that we have. I am working day to day to keep from getting scared of the intensity of it, the intimacy, the emotional vulnerability hitting so close to my divorce.

But hey, when it's right it's right. I've been reading about twin flames, soul mates, and what not, and well, this man seems to fit the bill. I'm hoping that by the time this book comes out, he will have already figured this out. I am grateful to the universe for meeting him, helping to mend our hearts at the same time.

We have both been through so much pain, and are truly still in the midst of it. Each day seems to draw forth a new conflict. His pain has literally manifested at his heart, through chronic heartburn and acid reflux after meals, something he's been suffering for years (since he was first married, but I have yet to point that out).

And when I'm with him, strangely, I often feel his pain in my own chest. Maybe it's a sympathy thing. I'd like to think we have travelled many lifetimes together, most probably as lovers because it's just too natural and familiar, and the pain I feel through him is pure compassion.

How do we heal this? Through presence, love. We have lain chest to chest and I have consciously sent my loving, healing thoughts to his heart chakra, with no expectations. After all, if it can't hurt, it can only help, right?

Meanwhile, back at the ranch, I spent last night consoling my little one, who has not seen her father in two weeks. At the end of a string of gut-wrenching sobs, she sniffled and said, in only the lisping way a small child can, 'My heart is bwoke.'

We had spent the afternoon doing yoga, at her suggestion. A playful kids' yoga, pretending we're animals and various things from nature, which all the poses are named after. It was so healing for both of us, different of course from the usual yoga I put out there for the broken hearted. But sometimes, you just need to play.

Her father, my ex-husband, went off the wagon after our face-to-face meeting, getting drunk and attempting to commit suicide, threatening this in front of the kids. He also called my reunion friend, when he was slurring his words, telling him to stay away from 'his wife'. He also tried to call my soul-mate friend, but he accidentally called a client instead. Eek.

This all should make me mad. Instead, it makes me very sad. I can't even imagine the pain he must be going through, and there's nothing I can do about it. I must forgive him, because he doesn't know what he is doing. I pray for him to get better, for my children's sake, because they, too, are now in a world of pain.

This morning we go to Olivia's therapist. How strange to have a therapist at age four. She is a grandmother, much in demand, with an office full of toys designed to help small children emote. Again, can't imagine it would hurt. She needs to express these feelings, and I feel like I need to do all I can to help her through this.

Brittany, so far, has refused therapy, has acted out, her face a wall of anguish and resentment. But last night was good. We went shopping, us three girls, our new family make-up. We sang bad Kelly Clarkson songs, and Olivia chased Brittany around the Adidas store, thinking, well, it is a running store. We were all present, for once. Those moments are just precious to me.

'Distance is the dagger in the heart of two lovers …'. So I spot this quote as I look up from my computer at a random coffeehouse where

I've selected to do some writing today. It is an apt quote for the day, despite the fact I have just left my lover after a quick bite to eat, a smooch goodbye, and off to our busy lives. But this yearning desire in my heart just won't go away, especially after another romantic night under the stars.

I want to grasp this happy feeling and not let it go, but I know better. This is good practice for *aparigraha*, non-grasping, yet another yogic limb. It is never enough. I want more and more and more of this man, to eat him up, contain him. I want to scream from the emotional intensity of this. Must breathe. Ramaramaramarama …

It's not like I don't have enough to keep my mind occupied, but when your heart has been broken, it wants to mend through more love. And again, this love must come from within before it can find wholeness through another.

Last night, my friend (I'll call him 'Wolff' just because it's funny) and I went to the lake on a whim, because it was a beautiful warm September evening and we were feeling giddy from drinking red wine at a Chamber of Commerce mixer. Wolff and I parked like teenagers, lay back in the back of his truck to gaze at the emerging stars, just high on life and each other, and made love for hours in the open air. I made a conscious decision to stay present, to not let my analytical mind ruin this night, to not worry about what my body looked like, that I was on my period (yes, yuck, but really, who cares?).

What does this have to do with yoga for the broken hearted, you ask? It is everything, I say. Yoga is pure presence. It is ultimate healing through acceptance, through forgiveness of your faults, compassion for the mistakes you've made in your frail humanness. It's about complete, fearless loving no matter what happens, whether you send this love to your partner, your kid, your dog, your neighbour, your enemy.

You are going to get hurt regardless – so what the heck? Life is all about hurt, about suffering, and how are you going to handle the pain? Are you going to curl up in a ball, to retreat into your turtle shell, or be a fierce warrior and break your own will until you surrender to the beautiful, magical force that pervades this world, that is as real as anything you see in the material world.

Last night I opened up some more, and it was a healing step in the right direction. Do I still yearn for Wolff? You betcha. But I will not act on this yearning for now. I will work with this energy, channelling it into my writing, my teaching, into moving forward, step by step. And again, I am happy with this process. It is a part of my becoming, of my blossoming into the real Michelle, the one that lies under the neurotic mess of my superficial personality. I know I'm much deeper than my problems, my perceived notion of what's wrong in my life. We all are.

CHAPTER 10
Journey Back Toward Love

'Love is all around
Step by step by step
Every day
Every way
Any day
The love will come.
Love is all around...
Nothing will diffuse that.'

OLIVIA HICKS (MY MUSE AT FOUR YEARS OLD)

This morning my daughter drew her feelings in her therapist's office. It was a beach scene, complete with sand, turquoise waves, a mermaid, and a little girl with a ponytail (a hook coming out of the top of her head). When the mermaid surfaced, the girl was happy, but when the mermaid went beneath the water, the girl was sad. Hmmmn ... doesn't really take a doctorate to figure out what's going on in my daughter's brain beneath the surface.

I understand the girl with the hook-looking ponytail ... after all, being a yoga teacher, my hair spends a lot of time up and off my face. But I am recognizing how much I compartmentalize my feelings into either 'good' or 'bad' and spend a lot of wasted time and energy avoiding the 'bad'. When I see Wolff, I feel happy. When he disappears, I am sad.

What's wrong with this picture? Well, my emotions are tied to an outcome, as well as to a person and circumstances outside myself. I can choose to be happy right now, with things exactly as they are. After all, I rationalize, I spent most of last night with him again, making love with a new-found fierceness and intensity that both surprises and scares me. It is a volatile feeling, a mixture of pain and pleasure that apparently needs to be released.

But this morning, I am tired and insecure, again. Why can't I be happy with things the way they are? Wolff is at work, for heaven's sake, and I am working and busy. I can't spend all my time making out, after all. This love craving is out of control, and I guess, like a food craving, instead of caving in I'm going to distract myself, so here I am writing. Good choice, Michelle.

Like the mermaid, I rise above the surface and sink below – I have to do this to be alive, to breathe! But I can choose to stay centred in the midst of it – that is yoga. Again, I remind myself: that is yoga.

When I can reach this state of loving calm, as I named it in my therapist's office, amazing things happen. In Patanjali's Yoga Sutras, it discusses mind-blowing magical 'powers' that one can attain through sustained meditation and various yoga techniques (not just the physical asanas). Some of them I experience, such as increased intuition and clairvoyance, the ability to see auras, and healing abilities, such as hot hands. It also describes what I would consider out-of-body experiences, calling it becoming 'invisible'.

This freaks out some of my teacher trainees, but it's fun to think about superpowers. Who wouldn't want to be like Superman or Wonderwoman? But it can seem awfully supernatural and freaky. I like to focus on the possibilities. If I were to hang out in a cave for a few decades, I'm sure I could learn all kinds of crazy stuff – but I'm not ready for that step yet (although a cave, today, sounds like a good idea).

But the psychic intuition has been really strong for me lately, especially at the end of class in *savasana* corpse pose, when my body and mind are not so restless, and messages and images enter my 'blank slate'.

Last night, for instance, after teaching two classes, I saw very clearly in my mind that my teacher trainee Claire, who was in class as a student, needed to 'look inside the box'. I have no idea what this meant, but the thought just would not go away. I didn't tell her after class, but later on when I was sitting in front of Wolff's house, waiting for him to get back from the grocery store, the thought returned and I couldn't shake it.

I called her, knowing she wasn't the type to think I'm a freak for this, and learned she was cleaning her closet earlier and had three boxes left to go through that had belonged to her parents, who were both deceased. She had been afraid to go through the boxes, feeling like she wasn't ready yet.

Well, as of this morning, she still hasn't 'looked in the box', but I know for sure there is something in there she should know about. I'm not sure if this message came from her mom and dad, or from somewhere else in the great beyond. Who cares? Sometimes these messages just come.

Of course, I'm not always able to apply these insights to my own life. Then again, I haven't asked lately. I think I'll do that right now – ask out loud to the powers that be that I have some peace, clarity, and abundance in my life. Do you hear that universe? Oh, and unconditional love, too, while I'm placing that order.

So, Claire looked in the box and found a card with a poem inside – something about the world being magical and full of possibilities when all doubts are banished … hmmn; could this be a message for her or for me, or for us all?

Tonight doesn't feel very magical. I do have doubts, fears, really. Wolff is out with an old girlfriend at an Elton John concert and I am jealous. I wish I wasn't, but I am. He told me a few days ago, excited at the opportunity, but later on when he heard in my voice that I had been crying, we had a big talk. You know the kind – the big talks.

First, he came over and fixed everything broken in my house – I guess that's how he shows his love, and that's a good thing, because my backed up pipes and busted doorbell were driving me nuts. Then we stood forehead to forehead and I was just brutally honest, that I was jealous and hurt, and even though I'm not ready for a commitment, so soon after a divorce, what we have is real and good and I don't want to date anyone else. He was honest, too, and it's obvious he's scared, and most guys when they get scared retreat.

At least he told me who he was going with. He could have easily lied. I appreciate this, but I'm still hurt – feels like someone just punched me. Then he got sick. I tried not to gloat, hoping he'd be too sick for his stupid 'date', and I did go out and buy him some medicine. He's still not feeling well, but well enough to go apparently, because he just sent me a picture of Elton on his picture phone.

Again, not sure what to do with this. If I go into my analytical mind, I could ask the question why he is texting me if he really likes this woman. I know he cares for me, he's just freaked out, as much as I am, about settling into a relationship that he's not ready for. I know this – I've been in this place before.

This time, I will choose to trust him. What other choice do I have? I will sit and breathe and send him my psychic messages of love and forgiveness, then read my child a story and go to bed before my chattering mind takes over again and I get neurotic.

After a rough night of tossing and turning, Wolff ended up taking me out on his parents' boat, which was incredible, and then the next evening we spent in my hot tub, doing a whole lot of unmentionable things (good, good things). Could this be the way to the divine? Those who study tantra believe so, but the strict *brahmacharyans* (celibacy seekers) would disagree. I think this could all be very intimate and awesome, as long as we (well me, really) don't get too attached to the pleasure part, just see it as a means to deep intimacy.

Of course, I can't tell Wolff this. Not sure if he's figured out yet that he's my soul mate, despite the obvious signs. We are in the part of our 'dance' where if we talk too much about what is going on between us he will freak out and run, because he's not ready for a 'relationship'. This is what all grown men do. And I'm not just being stereotypical. (All you women out there are laughing loudly now, aren't you? Or at least nodding your heads.)

So instead, I play it cool, telling him I'm awfully busy today (which I really am) and not calling him, but waiting for him to contact me. This is difficult, as my monkey mind is obsessed with him right now, fantasizing about the last few days, trying to grasp those moments with a tight fist. I need to just chill out and let him be for a while, let him want me. I know this, but it is hard. And yes, it makes my heart hurt.

In the meantime, my ex has reared his ugly head, and wants the kids this weekend. We go to court on Monday, so I decided it just wouldn't be a good idea until we see the judge and he can prove he won't get drunk, suicidal, and crazy (just a minor thing). This, too, is hard. I could really use a babysitter this weekend, as I have a big yoga workshop I'm hosting, but it's the best thing right now for my children, and if all goes well he'll stay sober and be able to take them the following weekend. Maybe I can go away for the weekend ... sigh.

According to my psychic, September 30 is supposed to be a big day for me, whatever that means. When you know the future, are you supposed to rearrange plans, like take the day off from work, or just leave things the way they are? When the same psychic told me my husband and I weren't meant to be together, I didn't want to hear it, and couldn't figure out if I needed to follow this or if it was a 'self-fulfilling prophecy', as in she told me it would happen so then I made it so by my own self-will.

Ultimately, she was right. She was able to tap into my marital un-bliss, which, looking back, really wasn't all that difficult. I can learn a lot about a person just by listening and paying attention to their body language. And since yoga teaches us to be present, to pay attention, to listen with all of our senses, it makes sense that yogis and yoginis could become, at the very least, extremely intuitive, and at best, really psychic.

As I write this, one of my yoga-teacher friends – whom we shall name Dandasana, because that's what he'd like to be called, and because it's funny since it means 'staff pose' – just called me and told me his new 'girlfriend' is mad at him because he got tired last night and didn't call her. Such a man.

I read him this last chapter, and told him women want to be called – a lot. Especially when they like you and are sleeping with you. If they don't like you, it could be misconstrued as stalking, which gets old and annoying, but if we like you, you need to call us.

This is yoga, too. Well, not really, but it's the truth.

More lessons. I am sitting with a bundle of emotions this morning. I was trying to quiet my mind in meditation at the ungodly hour of 5:00 a.m., when a strong voice in my head told me to get out of bed. Very quickly I tapped into a definite feeling of fear, and when I asked aloud where that fear was held in my body, it was right at my heart.

And the message came loud and clear – we have a choice whether to hold fear in our heart, which constricts, tightens, like a fist, or to open up in love, which feels absolutely liberating. Do we want to welcome pain or freedom? It is a choice, and it has nothing to do with other people or situations. Love is a way of being that is our God-given right; we just have to own it.

Wow. That's pretty powerful.

This week Wolfe (there's must be a reason why I want to spell it differently now, with a silent 'e' at the end, so I'm going to stick with that) and I had the most intense, the most intimate experience where I literally felt like a light went off in my brain, that something opened up, something really divine. Then we were interrupted abruptly, and something shut down in his eyes, and he couldn't recover. We had pure love for a moment, and then snap, it was replaced with pure fear. It was tangible. And sure enough, the next night he came over and we had another heartfelt talk, with him trying to explain (very poorly) how he has no room in his heart for emotions, it's not me it's him, yaddayaddayadda …

All summed up it came to: 'I'm scared, and I need space from this.'

He said some pretty hurtful stuff, and it took me a few days to gain some objectivity and recover. He was trying to push me away. I sat curled in a ball in the dark and cried the next day, hurting worse than anything in recent memory, even my divorce; and we went to court that same morning! But my heart isn't in my former marriage, and his is still stuck there for now. He is still in love with his ex-wife, even if he knows it's over and he doesn't want to be with her. He hasn't moved on, and I have.

Fast forward to a week later, and I have given him space, with a great deal of self-control I might add, and even went on a 'date' with a guy who was an emotional-enmeshment coach. He did a detachment process with me (these are the kinds of dates I have) so that I may gain some objectivity from Wolfe. Then Wolfe and I went on a road trip for three days and had a fantastic time.

You don't need the details (lots of driving, talking, out-of-this-world sex, dancing in a small town, eating, drinking red wine, more great sex, nature, etc.). But the point is, we were both able to remain in the present, enjoying each other's company without projecting too far into the future, without analyzing our relationship, without trying to jam the other person into our unrealistic expectations.

Of course, now I'm facing the re-entry into reality. I had to pick up my daughter from her father's house, learning he had grilled her with questions about Wolfe. These things I am going to have to face, one conflict at a time. But I was calm, and I am calm, and I know I can keep working at this, at accessing my centre and speaking my truth. This is my yoga. I am 'getting' it.

The *gunas*: In *The Bhagavad Gita* and many of the old scriptures out of India discuss three levels of a person's energetic personality, describing them almost as individual entities, although they often vacillate during different periods of a person's existence. The lowest level is *tamas*, or sloth, laziness. On the opposite end is *rajas*, or restlessness, an overly driven kind of energy. Somewhere in the middle lies *sattva*, the law of calm resourcefulness.

Although I aim for being sattvic, usually I tend more toward rajistic, which is OK since it's the easiest to transform with meditation. When I am tamasic, as I feel this wet and grey morning in October, it's tougher to pull out of my slump. I am fighting off a cold; knowing the stress I've been through must be contributing to my weakened immune system, I need the rest. So maybe I'm not so much lazy as not wanting to work right now. And I still feel restless.

Again, it is meditation that can bring us back to centre, and so I spent my morning meditating, despite my sore throat and headache, and now that the pain has eased (could it be that simple?) I am working, writing. Wolfe is pulling away from me, energetically (yet as I write this, my cell phone beeps at me that I missed his phone call, although he chose not to leave a message – at least he's thinking of me).

I wonder if men understand how when they pull away from us due to their fears of intimacy, how much it pulls a hole out of our hearts. I know he doesn't intend to do this. In fact, he continually says he doesn't want to hurt me, and I have no reason not to believe him. He is just in his own fear, his own pain, and I must respect his process.

At some level, I wonder if I'm not creating this space for myself, as I most definitely need it, too. I am having a quiet day, just getting out of my pyjamas late this afternoon, writing and resting and reading and meditating, talking with my girlfriends, just generally taking care of myself. I cancelled my massage, as I didn't want to make my pregnant therapist sick, but that's OK, because today I needed this resting place; maybe then I can regain a sattvic mind.

So where am I going in this saga? I set out to write a book about the process of yoga as healing the heart, a way of sitting with emotion, telling the truth about what's happening, and listening to the messages spirit sends us. Today I think I've found my happy ending, or at least I know where I am headed.

Yesterday I taught two morning yoga classes, the first beginners' class full of brand new students, so I gave my introductory briefing as to what yoga really is. That ultimately it means 'union', a coming together of body, mind, spirit, of true realization that we are all one, that we all suffer and don't want to, that we all seek joy (but go after this through passing sensory pleasures). And that once we are able to get our bodies healthy and get the restless energy out, once we are able to quiet the incessant chattering of the mind, we open to our divine inner self, and witness our authentic goodness, our light.

I am learning how to just put this out there for the new people. I used to be afraid they'd think it was a bunch of New Age mumbo jumbo, but now I just don't care. It's time people realize the truth of what yoga is, why it makes them feel the way it does. Why it works, and has for thousands of years.

So after putting that out there, I was feeling pretty good. I went on to pour wine at the Art, Wine and Chocolate Festival, volunteering for my girlfriend who is in charge of putting on the city's event. Of course, I poured a little for the people, a little for Michelle, a little for the people, a little more for Michelle, until I was completely lit, and I don't mean in a spiritual way.

Then along came the cute guy running for mayor, who showed me his sailboat and played guitar and sang to me and told me I blew his mind. Just guess what happened. And while it is happening, guess who I am thinking of, feeling as if I am cheating; yet he told me to do this, that we are dating, uncommitted, but I am just not good at this juggling of men, and I know for certain now my love for Wolfe is real.

Now, this morning, I am off to a festival of a different sort: a holistic healing fair where I rent a booth for the yoga studio. There are various psychics, aura readings, and the like, and I usually attend not for the business it brings me, but because I like to wander around and network with other spiritual healers. I am hearing the same messages, again and again, and this is why I know it is time to stop writing my story, as I have found a conclusion, and start explaining some yoga poses.

I am meant to put this book out to the world, know that it will be successful. I do not need to get a 'day job', I need to keep doing my work and the money will start coming fast and furious. At some point in the future, I also need to do a video, and this will involve work with children. Wolfe is indeed my soul mate, and he is scared of getting hurt, but ultimately soul mates 'don't go away'. And I'm meant to be with him this time around, in this lifetime.

My best piece of psychic wisdom came from where I least expected it. A pretty well-known clairvoyant from England was leading a talk on faith healing, and my own hands were getting really hot, and he asked if anyone was feeling it, and so I ended up healing another woman in the audience.

She then turned around to heal me as well, and turns out she does a lot of past-life regression work. She said she felt a lot of heartbreak around my heart and stomach chakras, that my mate and I have been through many betrayals in past lives; but this time will be different. This time we will be able to forgive and heal and love each other, and that it was just beautiful.

Wow.

So whether you believe in psychics or not really doesn't matter. This is what I know is true: I believe in love. I believe it is the only thing that really matters. I believe that no matter how much you've been through, you will keep hurting until you understand the lessons, and you will keep hurting until you find the inner strength to love again, to love some more, to love like your life depends on it, because it does.

Yoga means union, and union is love. Union is spirit, and that spirit resides in you. It doesn't go away, no matter what you've suffered. That suffering was necessary to bonk you over the head until you realize what's inside of you. If you don't want to suffer, learn how to really love. Stop resisting, and let go. Yoga is love.

CHAPTER II
Gentle Warm-ups

_____

Pranayama breath control:
ujjayi breath, victorious breath

Prana is both our breath and our life force. *Pranayama* is controlling the life force, and *ujjayi* breathing is a form of pranayama. Ujjayi means 'victorious', as it is about mastery over mind and body. At its most basic, ujjayi pranayama is deep, even, rhythmic breathing. Nothing more to remember than that. People try to make it way too complicated.

Start by listening to the sounds of your breathing, slowing it way, way down; focus on the exhale, as your inhale will always return as long as you are living. Grow the 'out' breath a little longer each time, and allow the 'in' breath to come back organically. Keep your lips together, and allow the breath to move in the back of your throat, generating heat inside the body. This heat – the kundalini flames generated from the pelvis – burns toxins in the body.

The audible sounds of the breath (as if it is sipped through a straw in the back of the throat) help to drown out any to-do lists, any distractions, and begin to draw attention inward, toward the true self. Ujjayi breath is loud, like the ocean. It is difficult to describe to a beginner, but after a whole lot of practising, your breathing will grow deeper and not give you a head rush, but give you new-found power and peace. Don't be shy with your breath.

Pranayama breath control is absolutely the heart of any yoga practice! If you find you're not breathing, you're probably stuck in your analytical, rigid mind. Breathe more; think less.

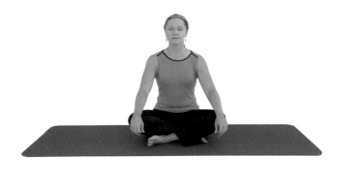

Neck and shoulder rolls: honouring boundaries

Begin by inhaling, tipping the head back, and exhaling, nodding the head forward, inhale back, exhale forward, chin to chest, nodding affirmation, nodding a big 'yes' to life, to love! Do this two–three times, then return your head to centre. Next take your chin to each shoulder, back and forth, turning your head as far as is comfortable, finding your 'edge' and working tension out of the neck and shoulders. Learn to honour your boundaries, as you say 'no' when appropriate. Return to a centre position.

Bring your shoulders up, back, away and down, as if swimming the backstroke through a beautiful, protected body of warm water, healing the rotator cuffs. Then change direction, drawing the shoulders forward, connecting breath with movement, realizing that yoga is now becoming a moving meditation, or meditation in motion.

Continue stilling the mind. As it wanders off into memories of the past (that have already happened and you can't do anything about), return your mind to centre. As it wanders into projections of the future, let go of expectations and judgements, as the future hasn't even happened yet. Stay present and in the now. Listen to the audible sounds of your breath.

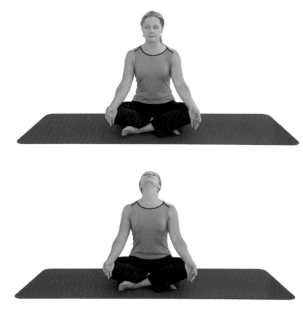

Child's pose: protection, cocooning

Move onto all fours, separate the knees, and draw the hips back with the palms on the floor in front of you, or rest your arms alongside your body, palms up, shoulders down. Either way is fine. Allow your heart to gently open and your pelvis to drop, releasing tension, doubts, fears and worries. Remember that this is a restorative pose, and you may return to it at any time in your practice. This is a particularly good pose to do in the first few days after a break up, or any loss, as you grieve. Spend some time here.

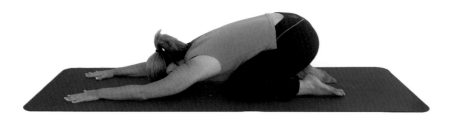

Cat/cow pose: massaging the central nervous system

Come back onto all fours, palms and knees on the floor, shoulders stacking the wrists, and beginning with a neutral spine (a flat back, not curved in either direction). Inhale, look up, fill the lungs, lifting the chest while dropping the belly like a saggy cow, then exhale, tuck the chin, arch the spine, stretching out the lower back like a cat. Repeat three–five times or until your lower back feels looser.

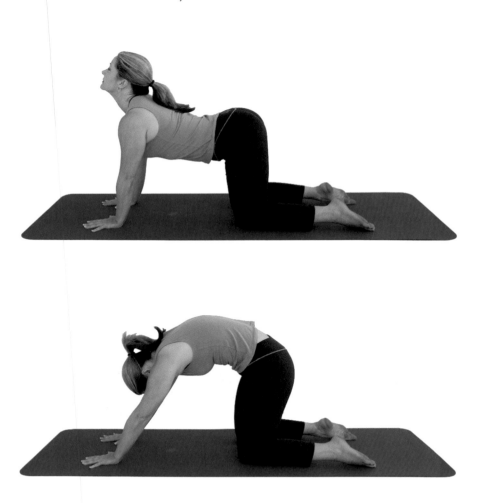

Downward-facing dog: home base

Exhale, push into your palms and lift your sit bones (literally 'the bones you sit on') high into downward-facing dog, feet hip-width apart. Look up to your navel or thighs, drawing your chest to your thighs, heels working gently toward the floor (eventually – these things take time). Remember to breathe deeply. You are working toward equanimity, or *uppeka* in Sanskrit, an even distribution in body, which also translates into evenness of mind and spirit.

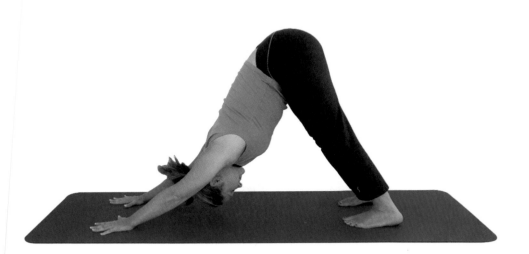

Rag doll forward bend: letting go of fear, anxiety, doubt

Inhale, walk, step or jump forward to the top of your mat, exhale, fold forward like a limp doll, taking hold of opposite elbows, softening your knees, and allowing your head, neck, and shoulders to hang gently. Maybe shake your head yes and then no, letting go of fear, anxiety, and doubts. Allow all of your troubles to just roll off your back.

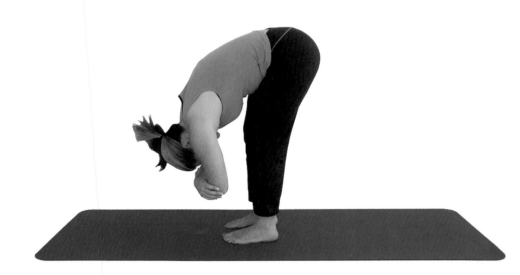

Mountain: building strength and hope

Separate your feet hip-distance apart and align your shoulders over your hips over your feet. Press all four corners of your feet into the earth below, and stand tall and strong like a mountain. Shoulders are back, spine is long, arms hang loosely. This is a foundational pose that will enable you to keep a tall posture throughout your practice.

Set an intention here or dedicate your practice, or even ask a question of the universe, paying attention to any images that come up for you. Be careful not to grasp onto these images; just take note, be grateful and let it go, knowing the lesson will come later when you are finished with your practice. If you are in (emotional) pain, if you are suffering, stand tall and connect with your majesty, again, just like a mountain. Visualize the mountain.

Sun salutes: devotion

Put your hands together, prayer-fashion (*samastitihi*, equal standing pose), inhale, then sweep your arms in a circle to meet overhead, looking up at your thumbs.

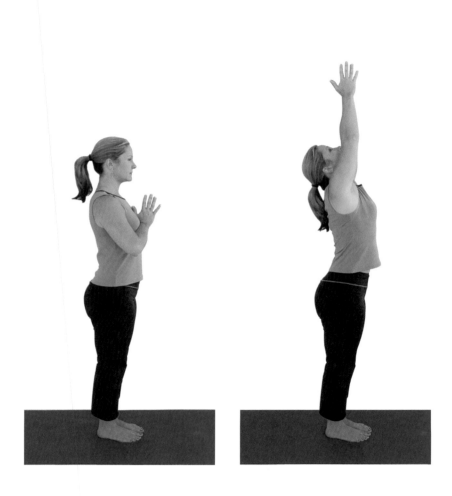

Exhale, swan dive forward toward your toes. Inhale, look up and lengthen your spine, fingertips to the floor.

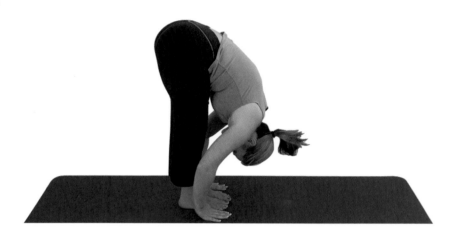

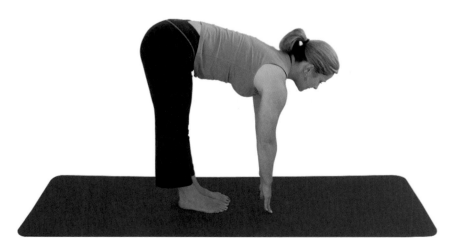

Exhale, put your hands flat on the floor, then step or jump back to a push-up position – *chaturanga dandasana* or plank pose. Bend your knees to the floor to modify, or lower your body from a high to a low push-up, hovering with your elbows hugged in close to your body.

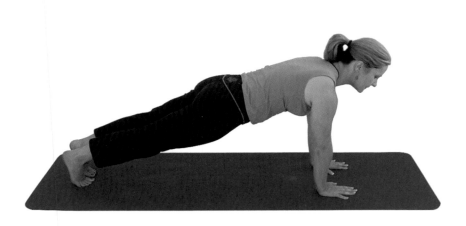

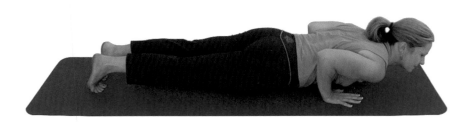

Inhale as you roll forward to straighten out your feet, then, with straight arms, lift the chest and heart, keeping your head up and shoulders back (upward-facing dog).

Exhale, push back into downward-facing dog, and hold for five breaths.

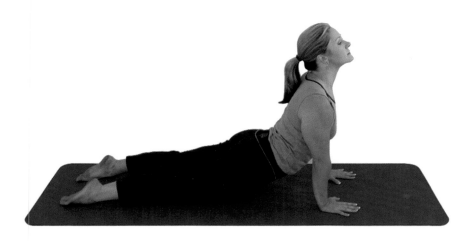

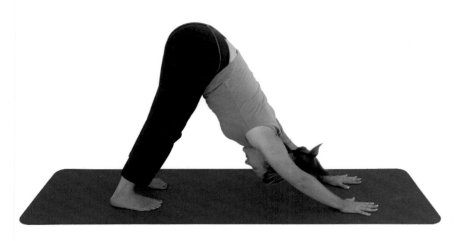

At the end of the fifth exhale, inhale and walk, step or jump to the top of your mat, and exhale, fold forward. Inhale, straighten up as you sweep your arms in a circle to meet overhead, palms together, then exhale, return to *samastitihi*, equal standing pose.

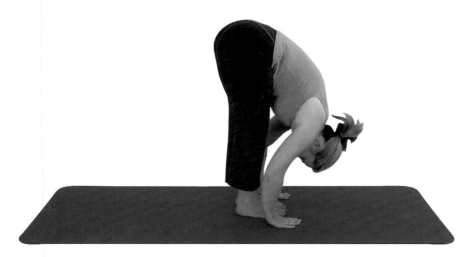

Repeat three–five times, keeping in mind how in ancient times this was done with a deep devotion, when people didn't know that the sun would return each day. Sun salutes warm up the body, increasing blood flow and circulation, improving flexibility and fanning the kundalini flames from the pelvis, generating heat that burns off toxins and impurities. This also serves to give you energy if it is lacking, or to work off excess anxiety if you are restless.

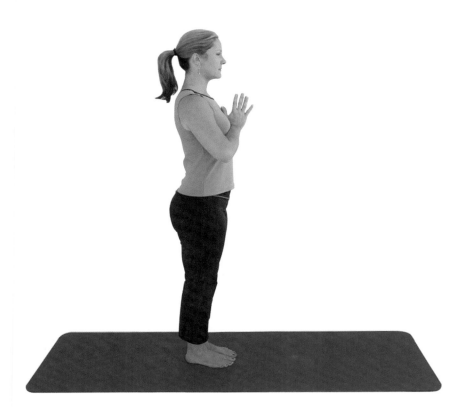

CHAPTER 12
Active Poses

Triangle: radiating inner light

Inhale, bend the knees, and open up to the right side of your mat with your feet three–four feet apart. Right toes point out; left toes turn in. Inhale, take your arms to a T, exhale, lean out to the right, reaching for your shin, ankle, or big toe (or to a block to modify). Extend (straighten) through the ribs, reaching up toward the sky with the left hand. Drishti focal point is your left thumb. (*Drishti* is a focal point for your eyes, which helps with balance and correct alignment, as well as stilling a wandering mind.) Spread your fingers and radiate your truth, your *satya*. What is your truth in this moment? Hips should be stacked, with the left hip moving back and the right hip moving forward. Consciously soften the left shoulder blade while strengthening the arms and engaging the legs. Repeat on the other side.

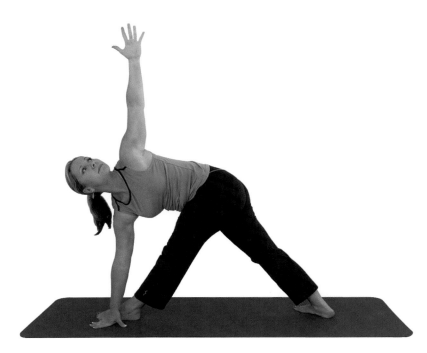

Revolved triangle: digesting change and new ideas

Pivot all the way to the other side, hands on hips, with both hips evenly facing forward. Again, feet should be three–four feet apart. Inhale, lift the left arm above your head, exhale, fold forward, inhale, lengthen the spine, moving the head away from the tailbone. Exhale, puff the belly out and spiral the chest to the right, placing your left hand on the floor and extending the right arm for the full pose. Drishti is the right thumb, or up at the ceiling if your hand remains on the hip to modify the pose. Pretend someone is behind you (or get a partner) pulling back on your quadriceps (front thigh muscles). Lengthen the spine on each inhale, and twist further into your pose on the exhale, finding your edge. Repeat on the other side.

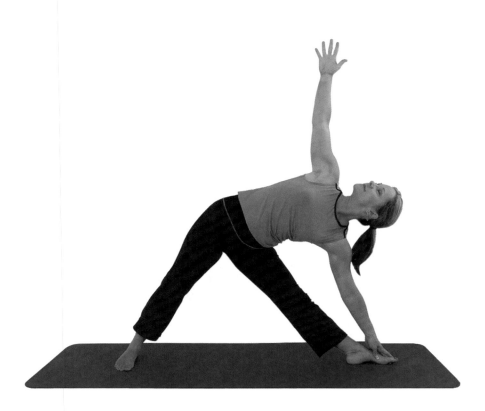

Mini prasarita series: opening the heart chakra

Bend your knees and open again to the right side of your mat, feet three–four feet apart and parallel to the edges of your mat, hands at your waist. Inhale, look up and lift your chest. Exhale, fold forward, and take your hands to your mat or a block to modify. Inhale, look up again and lengthen your spine; exhale, fold again, pointing the elbows behind you like a box, drawing your chest to your thighs. Shift your weight forward over your arches, until you feel a long stretch in your back hamstrings. Imagine all your fears and worries draining out of your brain and into mother Earth beneath you … she can handle it.

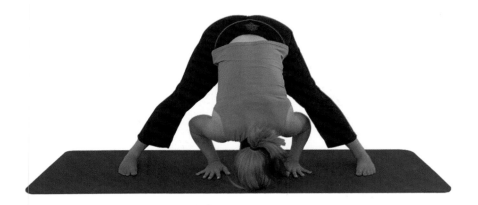

Inhale, look up, and exhale, take your hands to your hips. Inhale, come the rest of the way up to standing, and exhale; take your arms out to a side T. Take a moment to centre yourself, especially if you experience a little head rush. Draw your arms behind you, lacing your fingers and bringing your shoulder blades together. Inhale, look upward and lift your heart; exhale, bend forward, opening your heart chakra.

Ask internally where you may be holding back in this pose, and imagine filling your heart with self-love, compassion, and forgiveness. Soften your knees, and see if you can allow the natural forces of gravity to draw your arms ahead of you, opening you to more divine love than you can conceive. Hold this pose until you feel a sense of fulfilment and peace. Inhale, slowly come up with knees soft, and exhale, take your hands to your hips. Inhale, then step or jump back to the top of your mat.

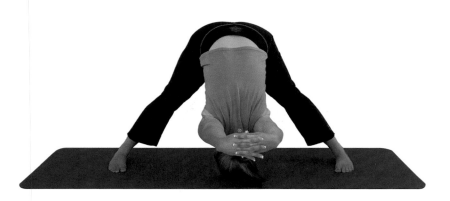

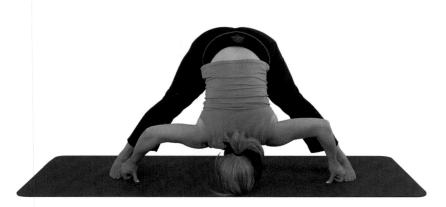

Tree: balance, yin/yang, masculine/feminine

Think about moving near a wall – even if it's just a psychological thing, it helps to have something solid nearby (to your side) in balance poses. Plant your left foot first, rooting your toes like tree roots, visualizing them growing deep into the ground. Bring your right foot inside your calf or upper thigh, below or above your knee, not at your kneecap. Clear your mind first of any distractions, and find a drishti focal point on the floor or wall, not on a person (as soon as that person twitches, it will be 'timber' for you!).

This pose is about 99% mental, 1% physical, so be sure to take your time emptying out your mind, and then bring your hands to your heart centre, in prayer fashion (*namaste* hands). If you are comfortable here, raise your arms above you and perhaps open up your 'tree branches' to the light, allowing that imaginary sunlight to pour through you, relaxing your shoulder blades down toward the pelvis, and curling your tailbone under. Take your hands back to your heart for a single breath, and release before turning to the other side.

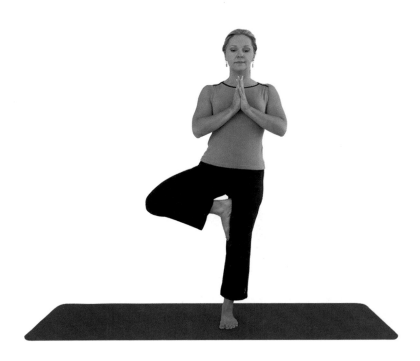

Utkatasana: owning your power

Move back to the top of your mat, in equal standing pose. (This is a starting point where you stand with equal weight on each foot, grounding all four corners of the foot into the earth, aligning shoulders over hips over knees, palms pressed together at the heart chakra.) Bend your knees, as if sitting back into a chair, and inhale, circle your arms above you. The full pose takes the palms together, but you may keep them open and parallel, to relax the shoulder blades down your back. If this is still too much, bring your hands to your hips. Again, scoop the tailbone under, and imagine the opposite forces at work in your body.

Inhale, sit a little deeper; exhale, reach a little higher. You are a thunderbolt of energy in this pose, so own your strength, your innermost power source. You are pure energy, pure spirit, building both physical strength and inner courage. You can make it through anything!

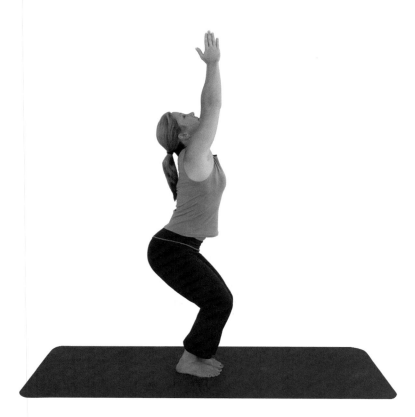

Warrior: strength, courage, endurance

From *utkatasana*, inhale and straighten your legs; exhale, dive forward toward your toes. Inhale, look up and lengthen your spine; exhale, take your palms to the mat and step or jump back into a push-up position (bent knees to modify). Exhale, lower your chest to just above the floor (hover if possible, just try not to 'kerplop'), and inhale, scoop up just your chest/heart, drawing your shoulders back and pressing through the tops of your feet into your mat. Quadriceps are engaged and active. Exhale, push into your palms and lift high into downward-facing dog.

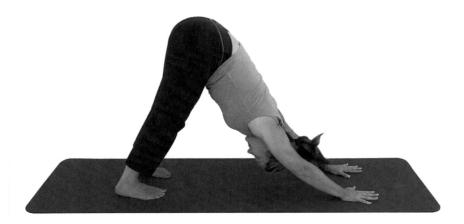

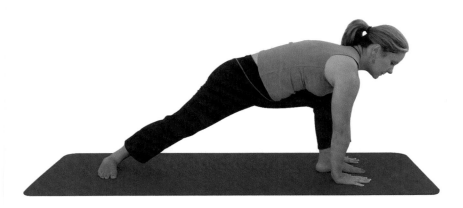

Inhale, turn your left heel inward so the foot is flat, and draw your right knee into your chest, moving it forward between the hands into a lunge, with the knee directly over the ankle. If this is tough for you (it takes a lot of core strength) try 'cheating' and using your right hand to push that calf all the way forward, and do be sure to stabilize the knee.

Inhale, and press through the back foot to come up, circling the arms above you with palms pressed and drishti as the thumbs, or modify with palms apart and just looking up if this bothers your neck at all. Lift from behind your heart, and feel the strength of a warrior, battling down the self-will. You are stronger than you know.

Inhale, straighten the front leg and pivot to the other side, repeating the same pose. After five–ten breaths, keeping your feet where they are, drop your arms out to a side T, in line with your feet, and open your hips and chest to the side of your mat. Turn to look over your front third finger, and be sure to keep your back arm lifted and strong, extending out to infinity. Perhaps take your palms up, and then down, imagining you are emptying out any suffering, any anger, frustration, disappointment, loneliness.

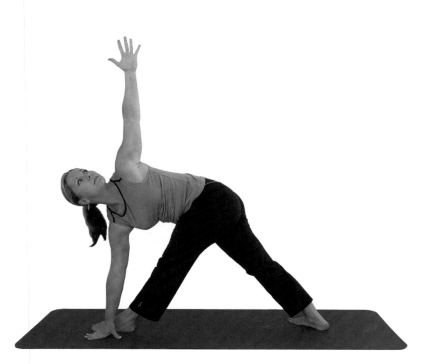

Inhale, and pivot your body to the other side, and this time, while taking the palms up and down, imagine filling the emptiness, the void, with love and light, faith and peace. Exhale, windmill your arms down to your mat, and cycle a mini-*vinyasa* (connecting the poses in flow), moving from *chaturanga dandasana* (push-up) into upward-facing dog, downward-facing dog, and then drop down into child's pose.

Take a few moments to check in with self, noticing any new sensations in the body without judgement, without labels. Just notice. Become an objective witness to your thoughts and emotions.

Yeah! We are almost half-way there …

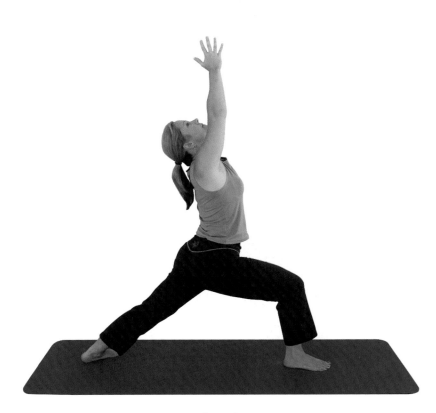

CHAPTER 13
Exploratory Poses

———

Pigeon pose: opening the hips, the seat of
our drama, releasing emotion

Inhale, draw your right knee forward, and take your left leg all the way
behind you, as far as you may take it. Sit to your right, perhaps on a
blanket or pillow to modify (especially if you have any knee issues),
and match up your right heel with your left hip bone. Square off your
hips toward the front of your mat, and lower to your forearms, or
eventually, all the way down to the floor.

Take some slow, deep breaths here. It may feel uncomfortable until
you allow the tension to melt away from the hips and pelvis, again a
place where we hold stress and emotion. If you are doing the pose
correctly, it should feel as if you have a fist in your right 'cheek', and I
don't mean the one in your face. Imagine that fist opening one finger
at a time with every breath you take, or picture a tight blossom opening
into a beautiful lotus flower.

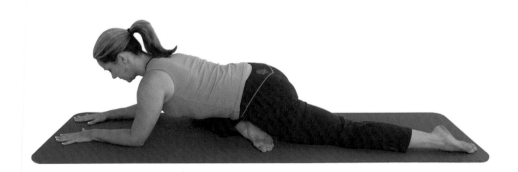

Pay attention to whatever feelings may surface here. It is normal to suddenly feel fear or anger or sadness. Try not to analyze these emotions, but feel safe enough to let them surface into the light of your awareness. Maybe say to yourself, 'Yeah, I feel sad' or 'I feel pissed off'. Sit with those feelings, however uncomfortable they make you feel in this moment.

The feelings themselves will not kill you. If you need to cry, so be it. People (men, too) cry in my classes all the time, and usually I don't notice, or if I do, I just know they need the release. If you don't know where that sadness or rage stems from, that's OK. You don't need a reason. Just feel it, and when the time feels right, see if you can just breathe and let it go.

Give yourself permission to release that emotion right out of your body, before it decides to manifest into some injury or illness. And please don't be embarrassed. There is absolutely no shame in this process. Let it go. Take as long as you need. Then make sure you do the same for your other side. Sit to your side and swing both feet forward (like you are break-dancing) and come into a seated position.

Staff pose: opening the chakras, 72,000 nadis or nerve channels

Extend your legs, with the energy moving out through the heels, flexing your feet (toes up), but keeping your heels on the floor. Bring your palms down beside you, fingers forward, and inhale, lift your shoulders up, back, away and then down, exhaling deeply. Inhale, lift through the crown of your head, and exhale, slight tuck to your chin.

Visualize the seven chakras as energy wheels ('chakra' simply means 'wheel' in Sanskrit), spinning the colours of the rainbow along your torso. As you breathe in each colour, pay attention to any sensations in the body, and linger in those places that seem tight or constricted until you free them up.

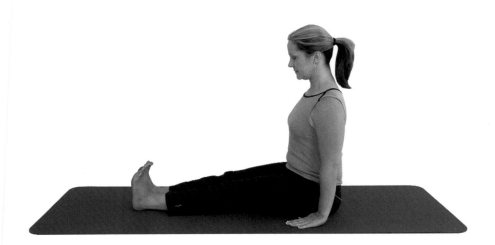

Red is at the base of your spine, orange in the lower belly, yellow in the solar plexus. These lower chakras have to do with the family of origin, with sexuality issues, with feelings in your 'gut'.

Green is the colour of the heart chakra, which of course is an important chakra for our purposes. How does it feel to breathe deeply into this area, filling it with a green healing light? What happens if you hold your breath in this pose, and draw out your exhale very slowly? What would happen if you released any pain in this chakra, and replaced it with pure love and light?

Now focus upward to the throat chakra, associated with the colour blue. This is the chakra of free speech, of self-expression. When your throat feels sore or tight, where are you holding back what you truly want to say? What are you afraid of?

Upward still is the colour indigo between the brows, the third eye or Christ consciousness or Krishna consciousness. It is a place for intuition or clarity. When focused on this area, it is common to actually 'see' a blue circle, sometimes surrounded by a golden light. This is where you may connect with your higher power. Pay close attention to what comes up for you in this circle.

Above the head lies the crown chakra, the royal colour purple. It is the chakra of wisdom, of unity, of enlightenment. Breathe up and down your chakras, like water moving through a fountain, and free up any blockages. How does this movement make you feel? Know that you may access this freedom at any time, just by bringing your awareness back to this moment.

Seated forward bend: relaxation

Inhale, circle your arms above you, and exhale, fold forward, reaching out to your shins, ankles, or eventually wrap your 'peace-sign' fingers around your big toes. If you can't reach your toes, try lassoing a strap or belt around your feet and hold lightly, guiding you into the pose, not using the strap as horse reins! Inhale, lengthen the spine (shoulders back) and exhale, fold deeper, gazing beyond your nose to your third eye, or out to the floor so you don't go cross-eyed.

Always lead with the sternum, taking care not to round the back and create strain. Even if it means you need to 'back off', it's better to work on correct alignment than to let your ego take control and hurt your back! You should feel this in your hamstrings in the back of your legs, and the act of folding forward calms the central nervous system. Do this pose any time you are stressed and need relaxing ... Hold for five–ten breaths or longer, depending on just how stressed out you really are! Exhale, release, and return to seated.

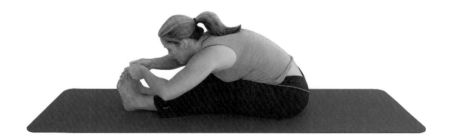

Marichyasana twist: aid digestion, relieve tension in lower back/neck/shoulders

Extend your left leg, and point your right knee toward the sky, your heel a fist's width from your inner thigh. Take your right hand behind you with the fingers pointed away. Inhale, lift your left arm, and exhale, draw your left elbow across your knee (or if that's too much, just hold your leg), gazing at a fixed point behind you.

Keeping your left foot flexed, inhale, lengthen up through the crown, puffing out your belly, and exhale, drawing your shoulders down your back toward the pelvis. Twist toward your gaze, not allowing your mind to wander. Imagine your body as a washcloth, and you are twisting out the toxins, twisting away any sadness. Repeat on the other side.

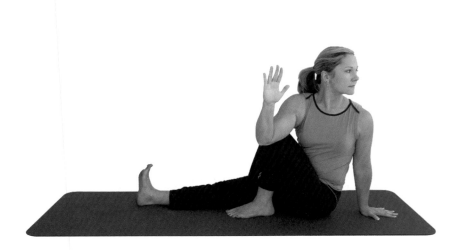

Boat: discover your core,
who you are beneath the roles you play

Bend your knees, with your hands behind your thighs. Close your eyes, and know that it is safe to go deep within your self. Inhale; puff your belly up, all the way to the diaphragm. Exhale, tuck the belly in and under, all the way to your spine, to the *uddiyana bandha*, the core. Inhale puffs out; exhale tucks in. Remember that your core is not just your physical core, although a strong abdominal core is essential to good back health and digestion; your core is also your centre of being, not what you do but who you truly are!

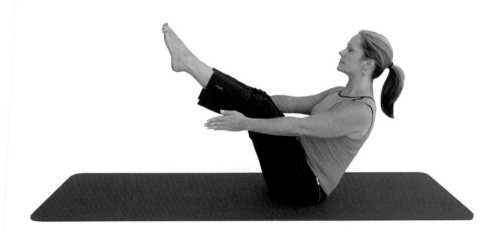

*Butterfly: represents change, opens hips with forgiveness,
compassion, strengthens the reproductive organs*

Bring your heels together in toward your body, opening up your feet
like a book. Close your eyes or turn your gaze inward. Inhale, imagine
you have a string lifting your crown toward the sky and lift your pelvic
floor (*mula bandha*), your kegel muscle. Exhale, allow that string, an
open channel, to run through your body, rooting your sit bones to the
earth below. Begin to lean forward with an erect spine. Allow light to
pour through that channel, healing those places you know need the
most healing. Never force the hips open. Allow the movement to
happen organically.

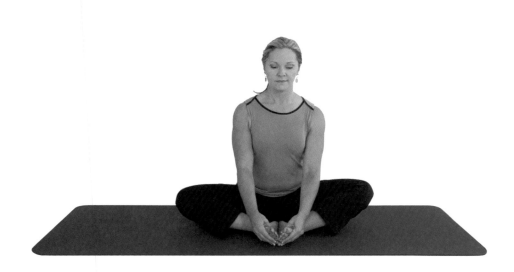

Bridge: opening the heart, connecting with something larger than your little self

Lie down on your back with your knees pointed up, heels near the body, feet hip-distance apart, palms facing down beside you. Press through the bottoms of your feet, lifting your pelvis and heart. Modify either by placing a block beneath your hips, or roll your shoulders underneath you, lacing your fingers and pressing the pinkies into your mat.

Engage your quadriceps, and keep your knees and feet parallel, not allowing your feet to splay out. Don't hold back here – go ahead and open your heart as wide as you can. Whatever heartbreak you have felt – and remember we have all experienced loss – what would happen if you let yourself open back up today? This pose bridges the self to the divine.

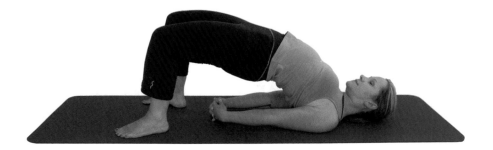

CHAPTER 14
Restorative Poses

Supported supta konasana (butterfly, lying down): resting the lower back, heart open

Again, lie down, bringing the soles of your feet together, allowing your knees to fall to the sides, with a pillow or rolled-up mat either lengthways under your back or under your knees. This time, allow your back to relax and release. Spend a few moments here, letting go.

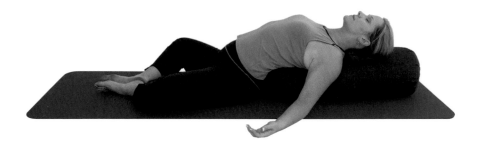

Legs up the wall pose: inversion to reverse the blood flow, inducing a peaceful state

Move your hips near a wall with your feet out to the sides, and roll your legs up toward the ceiling. If this causes any discomfort to the lower back, move away from the wall slightly. Keep your breathing slow and regulated, perhaps using an eye pillow if you have one to block out the outside world, practicing *pratyahara* (one of the eight limbs) or sensory withdrawal. Spend as much time as you can muster in this pose.

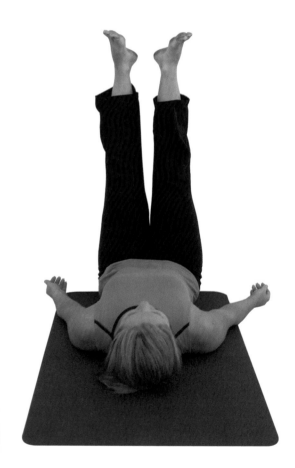

Savasana (corpse pose): final surrender, total acceptance, meditation, emptying the mind

Lie down on your back, extending your legs and allowing your feet to splay out to the sides. Arms are beside you, palms up and open, receptive and accepting. Breathe naturally now, eyes closed, and empty your mind completely. With your mind's eye, scan the body, releasing any leftover tension.

Start with the muscles of the face, smoothing the brows, unclenching your jaw, allowing your eyes to fall back in their sockets, your tongue falling back in the throat. Relax down through the neck and shoulders, down through the arms, paying extra attention to the hands. When your mind wanders, just bring your awareness back to the hands, and see if you can feel a healing heat, just by using your powerful mind/body connection.

Return to the torso, thanking all the internal organs in this region, working so hard for you, effortlessly, without you even trying. Bless your heart, your lungs, your intestines, your reproductive organs. Move your awareness into the bowl of your pelvis, further releasing any emotion, letting go of the drama. Move down through the legs: the quadriceps, the hamstrings, behind your kneecaps, down through the calves, and out through the bottoms of your feet and your toes.

Imagine a white or golden light passing through the whole of your body, all your fears and worries and anxieties draining deep into the floor, your thoughts becoming lighter than air, passing by like clouds in the sky. Let go of your 'to-do' lists, and if your mind projects into the future, realize that the future has not even happened yet, and the past is over. Be in the now, empty the mind, relax, surrender to what is and let go.

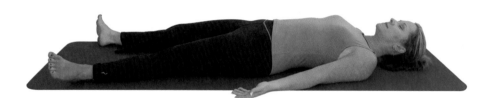

Endnotes

1 Geshe Michael Roach and Christie McNally, *The Essential Yoga Sutra: Ancient Wisdom for Your Yoga* (New York: Doubleday, 2005)
2 Eknath Easwaran, *The Bhagavad Gita* (Tomales, California: Nilgiri Press, 1998)
3 Eknath Easwaran, *The Bhagavad Gita* (Tomales, California: Nilgiri Press, 1998) p164

Acknowledgements

The quote from *The Bhagavad Gita*, translated by Eknath Easwaran, founder of the Blue Mountain Center of Meditation, copyright 1985; reprinted by permission of Nilgiri Press, P O Box 256, Tomales, CA 94971, www.easwaran.org.

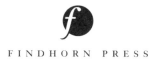

FINDHORN PRESS

Books, Card Sets,
CDs & DVDs
that inspire and uplift

For a complete catalogue,
please contact:

Findhorn Press Ltd
305a The Park, Findhorn
Forres IV36 3TE
Scotland, UK

Telephone +44-(0)1309-690582
Fax +44-(0)1309-690036
eMail info@findhornpress.com

or consult our catalogue online
(with secure order facility) on
www.findhornpress.com